Histoplasmosis

Protecting Workers at Risk

Steven W. Lenhart, CIH
Millie P. Schafer, PhD
Mitchell Singal, MD, MPH
Rana A. Hajjeh, MD

DEPARTMENT OF HEALTH AND HUMAN SERVICES
Centers for Disease Control and Prevention
National Institute for Occupational Safety and Health

National Center for Infectious Diseases

December 2004

ORDERING INFORMATION

To receive documents or more information about occupational safety and health topics, contact the National Institute for Occupational Safety and Health (NIOSH) at

NIOSH—Publications Dissemination
4676 Columbia Parkway
Cincinnati, OH 45226–1998

Telephone: 1–800–35–NIOSH (1–800–356–4674)
Fax: 1–513–533–8573
E-mail: pubstaff@cdc.gov

or visit the NIOSH Web site at www.cdc.gov/niosh

DHHS (NIOSH) Publication No. 2005–109 (supersedes 97–146)

Foreword

This booklet is a revised edition of the NIOSH document *Histoplasmosis: Protecting Workers at Risk*, which was originally published in September 1997. The updated information in this booklet will help readers understand what histoplasmosis is and recognize activities that may expose workers to the disease-causing fungus *Histoplasma capsulatum*. The booklet also informs readers about methods they can use to protect themselves and others from exposure.

Outbreaks of histoplasmosis have shared similar circumstances: People who did not know the health risks of breathing in the spores of *H. capsulatum* became ill and sometimes caused others nearby to become ill when they disturbed contaminated soil or accumulations of bird or bat manure. Because they were unaware of the hazard, they did not take protective measures that could have prevented illness.

This booklet will help prevent such exposures by serving as a guide for safety and health professionals, environmental consultants, supervisors, and others responsible for the safety and health of those working near material contaminated with *H. capsulatum*. Activities that pose a health risk to workers at these sites include disturbance of soil at an active or inactive bird roost or poultry house, excavation in regions where this fungus is endemic, and removal of bat or bird manure from buildings.

Local, State, and national public health professionals may also find this booklet useful for understanding the health risks of exposure to *H. capsulatum* so that they can provide guidance about work practices and personal protective equipment. The appendix consists of a fact sheet about histoplasmosis printed in English and Spanish. This fact sheet is intended to help educate workers and the general public about this disease. We urge employers, health agencies, unions, and cooperatives to distribute the fact sheet to all potentially exposed workers.

John Howard, M.D.
Director, National Institute for
   Occupational Safety and Health
Centers for Disease Control and Prevention

Authors and Acknowledgments

This booklet was written by Mr. Steven W. Lenhart, Dr. Millie P. Schafer, and Dr. Mitchell Singal, National Institute for Occupational Safety and Health (NIOSH), Centers for Disease Control and Prevention (CDC), and Dr. Rana A. Hajjeh, National Center for Infectious Diseases (NCID), also of CDC. Secretarial support was provided by Ms. Ellen Blythe. Ms. Priscilla Wopat, Spokane Research Laboratory, NIOSH, was the document's editor. Ms. Pauline Elliott of NIOSH, formatted the document. The cover design and respirator drawings were created by Mr. Richard A. Carlson. The histoplasmosis fact sheet was translated to Spanish by Dr. Veronica Herrera-Moreno and Dr. Tania Carreon-Valencia. The authors also extend gratitude to Dr. Donald L. Campbell, Ms. Teresa A. Seitz, Mr. Kenneth F. Martinez, and Ms. Dawn G. Tharr of NIOSH; Dr. Ted Pass II of Morehead State University; and Dr. Myat Htoo Razak for their encouragement and invaluable contributions to this work.

CONTENTS

Histoplasmosis
Protecting Workers at Risk

What is histoplasmosis?

Histoplasmosis is an infectious disease caused by inhaling the spores of a fungus called *Histoplasma capsulatum*. Histoplasmosis is not contagious; it cannot be transmitted from an infected person or animal to someone else.[1]

H. capsulatum is a dimorphic fungus, which means it has two forms.[2,3] It is a mold (mycelial phase) in soil at ambient temperatures, and after being inhaled by humans or animals, it produces a yeast phase when spores undergo genetic, biochemical, and physical alterations.[3] Spores of *H. capsulatum* are oval and have two sizes. Macroconidia (large spores) have diameters ranging from 8 to 15 micrometers (μm), and microconidia (small spores) range from 2 to 5 μm in diameter.[3] Yeast cells of *H. capsulatum* have oval to round shapes and diameters ranging from 1 to 5 μm.[3–5]

Histoplasmosis primarily affects a person's lungs, and its symptoms vary greatly. The vast majority of infected people are asymptomatic (have no apparent ill effects), or they experience symptoms so mild they do not seek medical attention and may not even realize that their illness was histoplasmosis.[6] If symptoms do occur, they will usually start within 3 to 17 days after exposure, with an average of 10 days.[1] Histoplasmosis can appear as a mild, flu-like respiratory illness and has a combination of symptoms, including malaise (a general ill feeling), fever, chest pain, dry or nonproductive cough, headache, loss of appetite, shortness of breath, joint and muscle pains, chills, and hoarseness.[1,3,6–8]

A chest X-ray of a person with acute pulmonary histoplamosis will commonly show a patchy pneumonitis, which eventually calcifies.[3]

Several years ago, pulmonary calcifications were thought to be associated with healed tuberculosis, when a person had actually had histoplasmosis instead. During the same period, individuals with histoplasmosis were admitted mistakenly to tuberculosis sanatoriums.[9] Unfortunately, some histoplasmosis patients acquired tuberculosis while residing in open wards with tuberculosis patients.[3]

Chronic lung disease due to histoplasmosis resembles tuberculosis and can worsen over months or years. Special antifungal medications are needed to arrest the disease.[1,5,6,10–12] The most severe and rarest form of this disease is disseminated histoplasmosis, which involves spreading of the fungus to other organs outside the lungs. Disseminated histoplasmosis is fatal if untreated,[1,13] but death can also occur in some patients even when medical treatment is received.[12] People with weakened immune systems are at the greatest risk for developing severe and disseminated histoplasmosis. Included in this high-risk group are persons with acquired immunodeficiency syndrome (AIDS) or cancer and persons receiving cancer chemotherapy; high-dose, long-term steroid therapy; or other immuno-suppressive drugs.[6,12,14–18]

A person who has had histoplasmosis can experience reinfection after reexposure to *H. capsulatum*. Persons with immunity to *H. capsulatum* who become reinfected will usually experience a heightened inflammatory response, but they will have a less severe illness of shorter duration than what resulted from the primary infection.[3,5]

Not to be confused with reinfection, *reactivation* of latent (inactive) histoplasmosis can occur in elderly and immunocompromised individuals years after infection by *H. capsulatum*.[2,5] The metabolic activity of dormant yeasts and the methods that enable a microorganism to escape elimination by a host's immune system are unknown.[19]

Impaired vision can develop in some people because of a rare condition called "presumed ocular histoplasmosis syndrome."[3,5,20–22] The factors causing this condition are poorly understood, and there is no scientific basis establishing *H. capsulatum* as its cause.[5] Results of laboratory tests suggest that presumed ocular histoplasmosis is associated with hypersensitivity to *H. capsulatum* and not from direct exposure of the eyes to the microorganism. What delayed events convert the condition from asymptomatic to symptomatic are also unknown.[23] This syndrome should not be confused with the involvement of the eye associated on rare occasions with disseminated histoplasmosis.[3,5] Because the lesions of presumed ocular histoplasmosis syndrome do not progress, treatment is not necessary; however, treatment is essential with active cases of histoplasmosis of the eye.[24]

How is histoplasmosis diagnosed?

Histoplasmosis can be diagnosed by identifying *H. capsulatum* in clinical samples of a symptomatic person's tissues or secretions, testing the patient's blood serum for antibodies to the microorganism, and testing urine, serum, or other body fluids for *H. capsulatum* antigen.[3] On occasion, diagnosis may require a transbronchial biopsy.[14]

Culturing of H. capsulatum

Culturing clinical specimens is a standard method of microbial identification, but the culturing process for isolating *H. capsulatum* is costly and time-consuming.[25] To complicate matters, positive results are seldom obtained during the acute stage of the illness, except from clinical specimens from patients with disseminated histoplasmosis.[6,12,14,25–27] However, research advances in polymerase chain reaction technology have resulted in methods that provide rapid, first-line detection and prospective identification of *H capsulatum* in clinical samples.[24–30]

Serologic tests

Serologic evidence is often the prime factor in the diagnosis of histoplasmosis.[31] Rapid and accurate determination of serologic test results depends on the proper collection, storage, and shipment of serum specimens. Thus, following guidelines established for these activities is essential.[31–33]

Because of their convenience, availability, and utility, the most widely accepted serologic tests are the immunodiffusion test and the complement-fixation test.[8,25–27] Serologic test results are useful when positive. However, sometimes test results are negative even when a person is sick with histoplasmosis, a situation that arises especially in patients with weakened immune systems.[6,14,26]

The immunodiffusion test qualitatively measures precipitating antibodies (H and M precipitin lines or bands) to concentrated histoplasmin.[8,14,34] While this test is more specific for histoplasmosis (i.e., a person who is not infected with *H. capsulatum* is unlikely to have a positive test result) than the complement-fixation test, it is less sensitive (i.e., someone who is acutely infected can have a negative test result).[8,14,25] Because the H band of the immunodiffusion test is usually present for only 4 to 6 weeks after exposure, it indicates active infection.[6,8,25] The M band is observed more frequently, appears soon after infection, and may persist up to 3 years after a patient recovers.[8,14]

The complement-fixation test, which measures antibodies to the intact yeast form and mycelial (histoplasmin) antigen, is more sensitive but less specific than the immunodiffusion test.[14] Complement-fixing antibodies may appear in 3 to 6 weeks (sometimes as early as 2 weeks[34]) following infection by *H. capsulatum*, and repeated tests will give positive results for months.[6,34] The results of complement-fixation tests are of greatest diagnostic usefulness when both acute and convalescent serum specimens can be obtained. A high titer (1:32 or higher) or a fourfold increase is indicative of active histoplasmosis.[8,26,27,34] Lower titers (1:8 or 1:16), although less specific, may also provide presumptive evidence of infection,[7,25] but they can also be measured in the serum of healthy persons from regions where histoplasmosis is endemic.[27] Antibody titers will gradually decline and eventually disappear months to years after a patient recovers.[6,8,25,34]

Detection of H. capsulatum antigen

A radioimmunoassay method can be used to measure *H. capsulatum* polysaccharide antigen (HPA) levels in samples of a patient's urine, serum, and other body fluids.[12,25,35,36] The test appears to meet the important need for a rapid and accurate method for early diagnosis of disseminated histoplasmosis, especially in patients with AIDS.[12,25,36] HPA is detected in body fluid samples of most patients with disseminated infection and in the urine and serum of 25% to 50% of those with less severe infections.[25]

Histoplasmin skin test

The manufacturing of diluted histoplasmin for skin testing was stopped in January, 2000. The skin testing reagents were still *unavailable* when these guidelines were updated in 2004. A person could learn from a histoplasmin skin test whether he or she had been previously infected by *H. capsulatum*. This test, similar to a tuberculin skin test, had been available at many physicians' offices and medical clinics. A histoplasmin skin test became positive 2 to 4 weeks after a person was infected by *H. capsulatum*, and repeated tests usually gave positive results for the rest of the person's life.[26] While histoplasmin skin test information was useful to epidemiologists, a positive skin test did not help

diagnose acute histoplasmosis, unless a previous skin test was known to have been negative.[6,8,14] A previous infection by *H. capsulatum* can provide partial protection against ill effects if a person is reinfected.[34] Since a positive skin test does not mean that a person is completely protected against ill effects,[34] appropriate exposure precautions should be taken regardless of a worker's skin-test status in the past.

Where are H. capsulatum spores found?

H. capsulatum grows in soils throughout the world.[2,14] In the United States, the fungus is endemic and the proportion of people infected by *H. capsulatum* is higher in central and eastern states, especially along the Ohio and Mississippi River valleys.[3,8,37] The fungus seems to grow best in soils having a high nitrogen content, especially those enriched with bird manure or bat droppings. The organism can be carried on the wings, feet, and beaks of birds and infect soil under roosting sites or manure accumulations inside or outside buildings. Active and inactive roosts of blackbirds (e.g., starlings, grackles, red-winged blackbirds, and cowbirds) have been found heavily contaminated by *H. capsulatum*.[34,38,50] Therefore, the soil in a stand of trees where blackbirds have roosted for 3 or more years should be suspected of being contaminated by the fungus.[42,51] Habitats of pigeons[38–40,52–54] and bats,[38,55–72] and poultry houses with dirt floors[38,73–78] have also been found contaminated by *H. capsulatum*.

On the other hand, fresh bird droppings on surfaces such as sidewalks and windowsills have not been shown to present a health risk for histoplasmosis because birds themselves do not appear to be infected by *H. capsulatum*.[34,79] Rather, bird manure is primarily a nutrient source for the growth of *H. capsulatum* already present in soil.[27] Unlike birds, bats can become infected with *H. capsulatum* and consequently can excrete the organism in their droppings.[27,62,65,80]

Increasing numbers of resident Canada geese in urban and suburban areas have caused concern about whether droppings and water contaminated by their droppings are possible sources of disease transmission to humans. As with exposures to the fresh droppings of other birds, exposures to goose droppings have not been shown to be a health risk for histoplasmosis. However, the human pathogens *Cryptosporidium*, *Giardia*, and *Campylobacter* have been found in Canada goose droppings.[81–83] The fecal-oral route is the primary route of ingesting pathogens that could cause infection and disease, notably diarrhea and gastroenteritis.[82] Thus, people working in areas frequented by Canada geese, such as ground maintenance workers at golf courses and parks, should take precautions to prevent hand-to-mouth contact with droppings.[81]

To learn whether soil or droppings are contaminated with *H. capsulatum* spores, samples must be collected and cultured. The culturing process involves inoculating mice with small portions of a sample, sacrificing the mice after 4 weeks, and streaking agar plates with portions of each mouse's liver and spleen.[38] Then for four more weeks, the plates are watched for the growth of *H. capsulatum*. Enough samples must be collected so that small but highly contaminated areas are not overlooked. On several occasions, *H. capsulatum* has not been recovered from any of the samples collected from material believed responsible for causing illness in people diagnosed from the results of clinical tests as having histoplasmosis.[39,40,61,74,84–86] Molecular techniques, such as polymerase chain reaction methods that produce results in days instead of weeks, may provide less costly and quicker methods of analyzing soil samples for *H. capsulatum*.[87]

Until a less expensive and more rapid method is available, testing field samples for *H. capsulatum* will be impractical in most situations. Consequently, when thorough testing is not done, the safest approach is to assume that the soil in regions where *H. capsulatum* is endemic and any accumulations of bat droppings or bird manure are contaminated with *H. capsulatum* and to take appropriate exposure precautions.

Who can get histoplasmosis and what jobs and activities put people at risk for exposure to *H. capsulatum* spores?

Anyone working at a job or present near activities where material contaminated with *H. capsulatum* becomes airborne can develop histoplasmosis if enough spores are inhaled. After an exposure, how ill a person becomes varies greatly and most likely depends on the number of spores inhaled and a person's age and susceptibility to the disease. The number of inhaled spores needed to cause disease is unknown. Generally, very few people will develop symptomatic disease after a low-level exposure to material contaminated with *H. capsulatum* spores. However, longer durations of exposure and exposure to higher concentrations of airborne contaminated material increase a person's risk of developing histoplasmosis.[5] Children younger than 2 years of age, persons with compromised immune systems, and older persons, in particular those with underlying illnesses such as diabetes and chronic lung disease, are at increased risk for developing symptomatic histoplasmosis.[3,4,14,88]

The U.S. Public Health Service (USPHS) and the Infectious Diseases Society of America (IDSA) have jointly published guidelines for the prevention of opportunistic infections in persons infected with the human immunodeficiency virus (HIV).[89] The USPHS/IDSA Prevention of Opportunistic Infections Working Group recommended that HIV-infected persons "should avoid activities known to be associated with increased risk (e.g., creating dust when working with surface soil; cleaning chicken coops that are heavily contaminated with droppings; disturbing soil beneath bird-roosting sites; cleaning, remodeling, or demolishing old buildings; and exploring caves)."[89] HIV-infected persons should consult their health care provider about appropriate exposure precautions that should be taken for any activity with a risk of exposure to *H. capsulatum*.

Below is a partial list of occupations and hobbies with risks for exposure to *H. capsulatum* spores. Appropriate exposure precautions should be taken by these people and others whenever contaminated soil, bat droppings, or bird manure is disturbed.

- Bridge inspector or painter[55,63,72,86]
- Chimney cleaner[66]
- Construction worker[12,57,58,67,85,90]
- Demolition worker[7,57,73]
- Farmer[7,12,74–77,86]
- Gardener[7,78,91]
- Heating and air-conditioning system installer or service person[8,61]
- Microbiology laboratory worker[23,53,64,86]
- Pest control worker
- Restorer of historic or abandoned buildings[61,64]
- Roofer[52]
- Spelunker (cave explorer)[56,59,60,68–71]

If someone who engages in these activities develops flu-like symptoms days or even weeks after disturbing material that might be contaminated with *H. capsulatum*, and the illness worsens rather than subsides after a few days, medical care should be sought and the health care provider informed about the exposure.

Outbreaks of histoplasmosis have occurred among people who were infected by *H. capsulatum* even though they had no part in the activities that caused contaminated material to become aerosolized.[39,52,92,93]

After a small group of students raked and swept a 20-year accumulation of dirt, leaves, and debris in a middle school's courtyard on Earth Day–1970,

nearly 400 people (mostly students) developed histoplasmosis.[92] The school's forced-air ventilation system, which had fresh air intakes in the courtyard, was implicated as being primarily responsible for spreading contaminated air throughout the school. Results of the outbreak investigation showed that a few students developed histoplasmosis despite being absent from school on the day when the courtyard was cleaned. This finding suggests that exposures to spore-contaminated dust continued for a day or more after cleaning of the courtyard was stopped.

During a histoplasmosis outbreak in 2001, 523 people (439 of them were students) met a laboratory-confirmed case definition of histoplasmosis following the rototilling of a 10-foot by 45-foot area of soil within a high school's courtyard.[93] Spore-contaminated air entered a wing of the school most likely through open windows that faced the courtyard and heating, ventilating, and air-conditioning systems that had fresh air intakes in the courtyard. As with the 1970 Earth Day outbreak, this study's findings also showed that a few persons were infected despite being absent from school on the day of the rototilling activity and the following day.

Should workers who might be exposed to *H. capsulatum* have pre-exposure skin or blood tests?

If a histoplasmin test was available again, workers at risk of exposure to *H. capsulatum* might learn useful information from skin testing. The results of skin testing would inform each worker of his or her status regarding either susceptibility to infection by *H. capsulatum* (a negative skin test) or partial protection against ill effects if reinfected (a positive skin test). However, a false-negative skin test result can be reported early in an infection or with persons with weakened immune systems.[6,8,14,26,34] A false-positive skin test can result from cross-reactions with antigens of certain other pathogenic fungi.[8,37] One drawback to routine pre-exposure skin testing is that a person with a positive skin test might incorrectly assume a false sense of security that he or she is completely protected against ill effects if reinfected. The work practices and personal protective equipment described in this booklet are expected to protect both skin-test positive and skin-test negative persons from excessive inhalation exposures to materials that might be contaminated with *H. capsulatum.*

Although a pre-exposure serum sample could be useful in determining whether a worker's post-exposure illness is histoplasmosis, routine collection and storage of serum specimens from workers is unnecessary and impractical in most work settings. Some employers, such as public health agencies and microbiology laboratories, have facilities for long-term storage of serum and do collect pre-exposure serum specimens from those employees who might be exposed to high-risk infectious agents. If a worker is to have blood drawn for this purpose and is to receive a histoplasmin skin test, the blood sample should be drawn first because the skin test may cause a positive complement-fixation test for up to 3 months and the appearance of the M band on an immunodiffusion test for *H. capsulatum.*[1,7,8,26]

What can be done to reduce exposures to *H. capsulatum*?

Excluding a colony of bats or a flock of birds from a building

Although a primary focus of this booklet is how to protect the health of workers cleaning up accumulated bat or bird manure, the best work practice is to prevent the accumulation of manure in the first place. Therefore, when a colony of bats or a flock of birds is discovered roosting in a building, immediate action should be taken to exclude the intruders by sealing all entry points. Any measure that might unnecessarily harm or kill a bat or bird should be avoided.

Before excluding a colony of bats or a flock of birds from a building, attention should be given to the possibility that flightless young may be present. In

the United States, this is an especially important consideration for bats from May through August.[94]

Ultrasonic devices and chemical repellents are ineffective for eliminating bats from a roosting area.[95] The most effective way of excluding bats from an occupied roost involves following five basic steps to identify and seal entry and exit points.[94] Because some bat species are so small that they can squeeze through an opening as small as the diameter of a dime,[94] even the smallest hole should be sealed. When openings are inaccessible, installing and maintaining lights in a roosting area will force bats to seek another daytime roosting site. Because of concerns for the welfare of evicted bats, constructing bat houses near former roosts has become a common practice.[94,96]

In some buildings, extensive bat exclusion measures may be more successful in the late fall or winter months after a colony has migrated to a warmer habitat or to another location for hibernation. In some regions of the United States, bats may not migrate, but rather will hibernate in the same building. Consequently, any work on a building that might disturb such a colony should be delayed until spring. Disturbing bats during hibernation is likely to result in their death.

Excluding birds from a building also involves blocking access to indoor roosts and nesting areas.[97] Because their food source is usually nearby, birds prevented from reentering a building will often complicate an exclusion by beginning to roost on window sills and ledges of the building or others nearby. Visual deterrents (e.g., balloons, flags, lights, and replicas of hawks and owls) and noises (e.g., gun shots, alarms, gas cannons, and fireworks) may scare birds away, but generally only temporarily.[97]

Nontoxic, chemical bird repellents are available as liquids, aerosols, and nondrying films and pastes. Disadvantages of these antiroosting materials are that some are messy and none are permanent. Even the most effective ones require periodic reapplication. More permanent repellents include mechanical antiroosting systems consisting of angled and porcupine wires made of stainless steel. These systems may require some occasional maintenance to clear nesting material or other debris from the wires.[97]

Pigeons can be controlled by capturing them in traps placed near their roosting, loafing, or feeding sites.[97] Shooting birds, using contact poisons, and baiting with poisoned food should be used as last resorts and should only be done by qualified pest control specialists. Using such methods to kill nuisance birds may also require a special permit.

Posting health risk warnings

If a colony of bats or a flock of birds is allowed to live in a building or a stand of trees, their manure will accumulate and create a health risk for anyone who enters the roosting area and disturbs the material. Once a roosting site has been discovered in a building, exclusion plans should be made, and the extent of contamination should be determined. When an accumulation of bat or bird manure is discovered in a building, removing the material is not always the next step. Simply leaving the material alone if it is in a location where no human activity is likely may be the best course of "action."

Areas known or suspected of being contaminated by *H. capsulatum*, such as bird roosts, attics, or even entire buildings that contain accumulations of bat or bird manure, should be posted with signs warning of the health risk. Each sign should provide the name and telephone number of a person to be contacted if there are questions about the area. In some situations, a fence may need to be built around a property or locks put on attic doors to prevent unsuspecting or unprotected individuals from entering.

Communicating health risks to workers

Before an activity is started that may disturb any material that might be contaminated by *H. capsulatum*,

workers should be informed in writing of the personal risk factors that increase an individual's chances of developing histoplasmosis. Such a written communication should include a warning that individuals with weakened immune systems are at the greatest risk of developing severe and disseminated histoplasmosis if they become infected. These people should seek advice from their health care provider about whether they should avoid exposure to materials that might be contaminated with *H. capsulatum*. The fact sheet in the appendix is one way of conveying information about histoplasmosis; it can be distributed to workers during their hazard communication training.

Controlling aerosolized dust when removing bat or bird manure from a building

The best way to prevent exposure to *H. capsulatum* spores is to avoid situations where material that might be contaminated can become aerosolized and subsequently inhaled. A brief inhalation exposure to highly contaminated dust may be all that is needed to cause infection and subsequent development of histoplasmosis. Therefore, work practices and dust control measures that eliminate or reduce dust generation during the removal of bat or bird manure from a building will also reduce risks of infection and subsequent development of disease. For example, instead of shoveling or sweeping dry, dusty material,[39] carefully wetting it with a water spray can reduce the amount of dust aerosolized during an activity. Adding a surfactant or wetting agent to the water might reduce further the amount of aerosolized dust. Once the material is wetted, it can be collected in double, heavy-duty plastic bags, a 55-gallon drum, or some other secure container for immediate disposal. An alternative method is use of an industrial vacuum cleaner with a high-efficiency filter to "bag" contaminated material. Truck-mounted or trailer-mounted vacuum systems are recommended for buildings with large accumulations of bat or bird manure. These high-volume systems can remove tons of contaminated material in a short period. Using long, large-diameter hoses, such a system can also remove contaminated material located several stories above its waste hopper. This advantage eliminates the risk of dust exposure that can happen when bags tear accidentally or containers break during their transfer to the ground.

The removal of all material that might be contaminated by *H. capsulatum* from a building and immediate waste disposal will eliminate any further risk that someone might be exposed to aerosolized spores. Air sampling, surface sampling, or the use of any other method intended to confirm that no infectious agents remain following removal of bat or bird manure is unnecessary in most cases. However, before a removal activity is considered finished, the cleaned area should be inspected visually to ensure that no residual dust or debris remains.

Disinfecting contaminated material

Disinfectants have occasionally been used to treat contaminated soil and accumulations of bat manure when removal was impractical or as a precaution before a removal process was started.[41,48–50,61,67] To date, formaldehyde solutions have been the only disinfectants proven to be effective for decontaminating soil containing *H. capsulatum*.[41,48–50] Exposures to formaldehyde through ingestion, inhalation, and skin and eye contact can cause a variety of adverse health effects.[98] Several years ago, applicators exposed to formaldehyde during soil disinfection activities reported burning eyes and mucous membrane irritation.[48] Workers at another site experienced nausea and vomiting.[41]

Today, although a number of EPA-registered fungicidal products contain formaldehyde, none of them is registered for use as a soil disinfectant. Thus, using a formaldehyde containing product to disinfect soil would be inappropriate. Furthermore, there is no product or chemical that is registered by the EPA that has the specific claim of being effective against *H. capsulatum*. A manufacturer of a product claiming to disinfect soil contaminated with *H. capsulatum* will have to meet the EPA's regula-

tory requirements and complete the registration process.

Should an EPA-registered product become available to disinfect land contaminated by *H. capsulatum*, measures should be taken to ensure that the disinfectant penetrates deeply enough to contact all the soil containing *H. capsulatum*. While *H. capsulatum* was found in a blackbird roost at a depth of more than 12 inches,[99] soil saturation to a depth of 6 to 8 inches will be sufficient for most disinfectant applications.[38,48] To evaluate a disinfectant's effectiveness, soil samples should be collected before and after an application and analyzed for *H. capsulatum*. The appropriate number of samples to be collected will vary depending upon the size of the property.[38,100] Each sampling location should be flagged or marked in a way that will ensure that the same locations will be sampled after application of the disinfectant. A map of the treated area showing the approximate location of each sampling site will also be useful in the event flags or markings are lost. After a disinfectant's effectiveness has been documented—more than one application may be necessary—additional tests for *H. capsulatum* should be done periodically if the land remains idle.

Disposing of waste

Any material that might be contaminated with *H. capsulatum* that is removed from a work site should be disposed of or decontaminated properly and safely and not merely moved to another area where it could still be a health hazard. Before an activity is started, the quantity of material to be removed should be estimated. (If the approximate volume of dry bat or bird manure in a building is known, the approximate weight can be calculated using a conversion factor of 40 pounds per cubic foot.) Requirements established by local and state authorities for the removal, transportation, and disposal of contaminated material should be followed. Arrangements should be made with a landfill operator concerning the quantity of material to be disposed of, the dates when the material will be delivered, and the disposal location. If local or state landfill regulations define material contaminated with *H. capsulatum* to be infectious waste, incineration or another decontamination method may also be required.

Controlling aerosolized dust during construction, excavation, and demolition

Dusts containing *H. capsulatum* spores can be aerosolized during construction, excavation, or demolition. Once airborne, spores can be carried easily by wind currents over long distances. Such contaminated airborne dusts can cause infections not only in persons at a work site, but also in others nearby. Such activities were suggested as the causes of the three largest outbreaks of histoplasmosis ever recorded. All three outbreaks took place in Indianapolis, Indiana.[25,85,88,101] During the first outbreak, in the fall of 1978 and spring of 1979, an estimated 120,000 people were infected, and 15 people died. The second outbreak, in 1980, was similar to the first in the number of people affected. AIDS patients accounted for nearly 50% of culture-proven cases during the third outbreak, which began in 1988 and lasted until 1993.[101]

Water sprays or other dust suppression techniques should be used to reduce the amount of dust aerosolized during construction, excavation, or demolition in regions where *H. capsulatum* is endemic. During windy periods or other times when typical dust suppression techniques are ineffective, earthmoving activities should be interrupted. All earthmoving equipment (e.g., bulldozers, trucks, and front-end loaders) should have cabs with air-conditioning (if available) to protect their operators. Air filters on air-conditioners should be inspected on a regular schedule and cleaned or replaced as needed. During filter cleaning or replacement of exceptionally dusty air filters, respiratory protection should be worn by the maintenance person if there is a potential for the dust to be aerosolized. Beds of all trucks carrying dirt or debris from a work site should be covered, and all trucks should pass through a wash station before leaving the site. When at a dump site, a truck operator should ensure that all individuals in the vicinity are in an area

where they will not be exposed to dust aerosolized while the truck is emptied.

Water sprays and other suppression techniques may not be enough to control dust aerosolized during demolition of a building or other structure. Consequently, removal of accumulations of bird or bat manure before demolition may be necessary in some situations. Factors affecting decisions about pre-demolition removal of such accumulations include the quantity and locations of the material, the structural integrity or soundness of the building, weather conditions, proximity of the building to other buildings and structures, and whether nearby buildings are occupied by persons who may be at increased risk for developing symptomatic histoplasmosis (e.g., schools, day-care facilities, hospitals, clinics, jails, and prisons).

City or county governments in regions where *H. capsulatum* is endemic should establish and enforce regulations concerning work practices that will control dust aerosolization at construction, excavation, and demolition sites. However, even in regions where *H. capsulatum* is not considered endemic, dust aerosolized during work activities in bird roosts has also resulted in outbreaks of histoplasmosis.[40,45] Consequently, regardless of whether a work site is in an endemic region, precautions should be taken at active and inactive bird roosts to prevent dust aerosolization.

Wearing personal protective equipment

Because work practices and dust control measures to reduce worker exposures to *H. capsulatum* have not been fully evaluated, using personal protective equipment is still necessary during some activities. During removal of an accumulation of bat or bird manure from an enclosed area such as an attic, dust control measures should be used, but wearing a NIOSH-approved respirator and other items of personal protective equipment is also recommended to reduce further the risk of *H. capsulatum* exposure.

For some jobs involving exposures to airborne dusts, working conditions have changed little over the years despite improvements in other aspects of the industry. For example, inhalation of dust aerosolized from the dirt floors of chicken coops that contained *H. capsulatum* spores was reported more than 40 years ago as the cause of clinical cases of histoplasmosis in workers.[73–77] As the poultry industry has grown, the old-style chicken coop has been replaced by larger housing facilities. In the United States in 2002, approximately 82,400 farms produced eggs or poultry including layers, pullets, broilers, turkeys, ducks, and geese.[102] However, the floors of most poultry houses are still dirt covered and provide an excellent medium for the growth of *H. capsulatum*. Ventilation systems in poultry houses are not primarily intended to reduce poultry workers' exposures to aerosolized dust, and dust measurements made during growing and catching chickens show that inhalation exposures of poultry workers to dust can be excessive.[103] Since ventilation systems designed especially to reduce airborne dust to "safe" levels in poultry houses would likely be economically and mechanically impractical, wearing a respirator is probably the most feasible method for protecting poultry workers.

Recommendations for selecting respirators to protect workers against inhalation exposures to airborne dust and *H. capsulatum* are described next. Following that, recommendations for personal protective equipment other than respirators are provided.

What are the advantages and disadvantages of various kinds of respirators for protecting workers against exposure to *H. capsulatum*?

Assigned protection factors

Respirators provide varying levels of protection, and people have developed histoplasmosis after disturbing material contaminated with *H. capsulatum* despite wearing either a respirator or a mask that they assumed would protect them.[60,71,104] Such unfortunate events demonstrate that when a respirator is needed, it must be carefully selected with an understanding of the circumstances associated with exposure to an airborne contaminant and the capabilities and limitations of the various kinds of respirators.

Because respirators provide different levels of protection, they are divided into classes, and each respirator class has been assigned a protection factor to help compare its protective capabilities with other respirator classes. An assigned protection factor is a unitless number determined statistically from a set of experimental or workplace data. This factor is the minimum level of protection expected for a substantial proportion (usually 95%) of properly fitted and trained respirator users.[105]

When the effectiveness of a respirator is evaluated in a workplace, a protection factor is calculated for each respirator wearer and respirator combination by dividing the air concentration of a challenge agent by the air concentration of that agent inside the respirator wearer's facepiece, hood, or helmet. For example, if air sampling measurements show equal concentrations of a contaminant inside and outside a respirator wearer's facepiece, then the respirator provided no protection, and a protection factor of 1 would be calculated. Likewise, a protection factor of 5 means that a respirator wearer was exposed to one-fifth (20%) of the air concentration to which he or she would have been exposed if a respirator had not been used, a reduction of 80%. Similarly, a protection factor of 10 represents a one-tenth (10%) exposure (a 90% reduction), 50 represents a one-fiftieth (2%) exposure (a 98% reduction), and so on.

The assigned protection factors of respirators available for protecting workers against exposures to airborne materials contaminated with *H. capsulatum* range from 10 to 10,000.[106,107,108] Disposable respirators and elastomeric half-facepiece respirators represent the low end of the protection-factor scale. Self-contained breathing apparatuses operated in the pressure-demand mode, represent the high end. Within this range is a variety of negative-pressure, powered air-purifying, and supplied-air respirators that are available with half-facepiece, full face-piece, loose-fitting facepiece, hood, or helmet. Later in this section, the advantages and disadvantages of these various respirators are described.

Respirator selection

Before the specific types of respirators are described, it is important to understand the information that is usually needed to select a respirator for a particular activity.

The hazard ratio method, or the industrial hygiene method, is a quantitative method used most commonly to select respirators for noninfectious aerosols, gases, and vapors. Using this method requires estimates of the air concentrations of a contaminant measured during a person's work activities and knowledge of the established (or recommended) occupational exposure limits of that contaminant. A minimum level of respiratory protection is calculated by dividing the highest air concentration measurement by the most protective occupational exposure limit of the contaminant. A respirator from the respirator class having an assigned protection factor equal to or exceeding this value would then be selected. For example, assume a set of air samples collected during a particular job resulted in exposure estimates ranging from 8 to 50 milligrams per cubic meter (mg/m^3) of sampled air for a contaminant having occupational exposure limits of 5 mg/m^3 and 10 mg/m^3. Given this information, a respirator with an assigned protection factor of at least 10 (50 mg/m^3 ÷ 5 mg/m^3 = 10) should be selected. However, applying the hazard ratio method to respirator selection decisions for infectious aerosols is difficult and often impossible.[109]

Unfortunately, published air sampling data on *H. capsulatum* spores are either outdated or too limited,[68–70,76,80,110,111] and no numerical exposure limit exists for *H. capsulatum*. In situations such as this, when the important data needed for the hazard ratio method are either uncertain or unavailable, the expert opinion method is usually used.[109] This method is a qualitative approach to making decisions about respirators based on the subjective professional judgment of one or more experts. Respirator selection is made after considering the characteristics of job activities that are recognized or anticipated to involve risks of exposure to airborne contaminants; consideration of the properties of the specific agent involved and health effects of overexposure; and knowledge of the assigned protection factors, advantages, and disadvantages of various respirators.[109] In this application of the expert opinion method, categorical risk estimates were developed with the levels of recommended respiratory protection increasing as the perceived levels of exposure increased.[109]

The following respirator selection information describes classes of respirators in order of increasing assigned protection factors. The assigned protection factors used here are from Table 1 of the *NIOSH Respirator Selection Logic*.[106] Respirators that should be worn during work activities involving exposures to spore-contaminated airborne dusts range from disposable, filtering facepiece respirators for low-risk situations (e.g., site surveys of bird roosts) to full-facepiece, powered air-purifying respirators for extremely dusty work (e.g., removing accumulated bird or bat manure from an enclosed area such as an attic).

Regardless of which respirator is selected, the device should be NIOSH-certified and used in the context of a respiratory protection program. Important components of such a program are facepiece fit-testing, respirator maintenance, user training, medical evaluation of users, respiratory protection program evaluation, and recordkeeping.[112,113]

Disposable and elastomeric, half-facepiece, air-purifying respirators (assigned protection factor: 10)

A half-facepiece respirator covers the wearer's nose and mouth. Because inhalation creates a slight negative pressure inside the facepiece of non-powered, air-purifying respirators with respect to outside, these respirators are also called negative-pressure

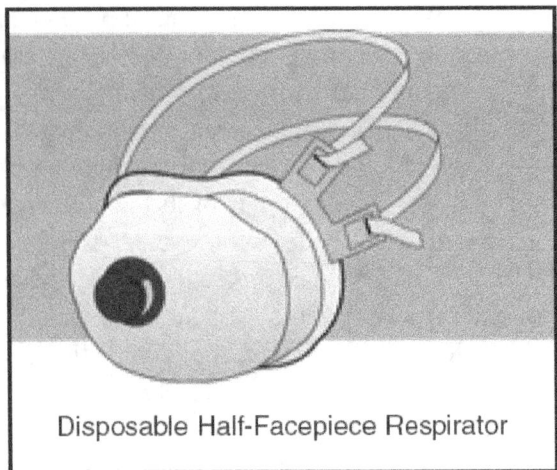

Disposable Half-Facepiece Respirator

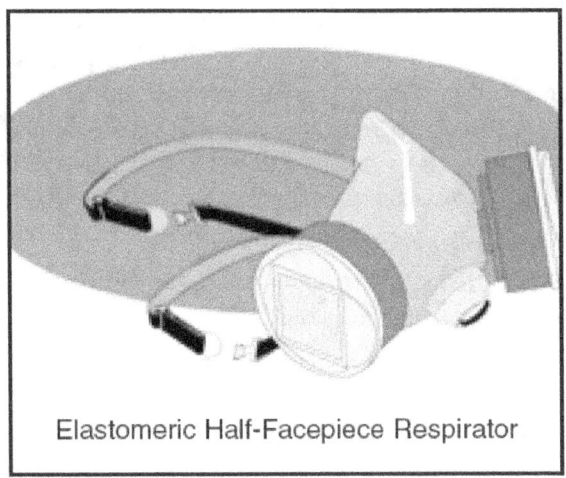

Elastomeric Half-Facepiece Respirator

respirators. During inhalation, contaminated air can easily enter the facepiece of a negative-pressure respirator at gaps between the facepiece and the respirator wearer's face. Therefore, a complete face-to-facepiece seal is essential for good protection. The findings of a study to evaluate faceseal leaks of an elastomeric half-facepiece respirator showed that 89% of the leaks occurred at the nose or chin or were multiple leaks that included these locations.[114] Facial hair (even the stubble of a few days' growth), absence of one or both dentures, and deep facial scars can also prevent a complete seal.

Whereas elastomeric half-facepiece respirators consist of a reusable elastomeric or rubber facepiece and replaceable filters, most disposable respirators are filtering facepieces in which the facepiece is the dust filter. Disposable respirators and replaceable filters can be used until they are difficult to breathe through, damaged, or malodorous.

A disadvantage of any negative-pressure, air-purifying respirator is that resistance to inhalation increases as the filters load with dust. For disposable respirators without exhalation valves, filter loading increases resistance during exhalation as well as inhalation. This effect, combined with the warm, moist air inside the facepiece, is so uncomfortable for some people that they do not wear a respirator as frequently as they should, or they stop wearing one entirely.

As of July 10, 1995, NIOSH began certification of negative-pressure, air-purifying particulate filters under new regulations (42 CFR Part 84).[115] All particulate-filtering respirators certified by NIOSH under previous regulations (30 CFR Part 11) were no longer sold after July 10, 1998, and only Part 84 particulate respirators are now available. Part 84 particulate respirators have the prefix TC-84A. Part 84 particulate filters are divided into nine classes, and filters from any class can be selected for protection against inhalation of *H. capsulatum* spores. A filter's class (e.g., N-95) and "NIOSH" are marked on the facepiece, exhalation valve cover, or head straps of disposable respirators, and on filter cartridges and cartridge boxes.

Although Part 84 improved the requirements for particulate filters, the facepiece fitting characteristics of all particulate respirators became exempt from evaluation as a condition of NIOSH certification.[116] Thus, only respirators with good fitting characteristics should be purchased, and it is essential that workers are assigned respirators based on the results of facepiece fit-testing. To aid in the selection of filtering facepiece respirators for fit testing, studies have been published on the fitting characteristics of some of them.[116,117]

The type of head straps on the various disposable and elastomeric half-facepiece respirators is an important but frequently overlooked consideration.

Head strap tension is important for achieving a complete face-to-facepiece seal without sacrificing comfort. Elastomeric facepieces have adjustable straps, which should allow a respirator wearer to make a complete, yet comfortable, facepiece seal. On the other hand, not all disposable respirators have adjustable straps; some simply have fixed-length elastic bands. Most disposable respirators certified under Part 84, do not have adjustable straps, only elastic bands. Research has not been done to evaluate whether the facepiece fits of respirators with adjustable straps differ significantly from those of respirators with elastic bands. However, a respirator user should be aware that the fit and comfort of a disposable respirator with elastic bands might differ from one with adjustable straps.

In dusty conditions, repeated exposure of the eyes to dust increases the risk for injury and disease. Most dust particles entering a person's eyes will be washed out by tears, but some particles can be retained, particularly within the margin of the upper eyelid. Depending on their size, shape, and composition, these particles can become embedded in the surface of the cornea or sclera, where they cause irritation and then reddening of the surface. If not removed, such particles may produce eye infections.[118] Therefore, a half-facepiece respirator is a poor choice for use in dusty conditions. While wearing eyecup goggles may provide some eye protection, they are not airtight and do not completely prevent dust exposure. Furthermore, goggles may interfere with a respirator's fit. For these reasons, a full-facepiece respirator is a better alternative when a person's eyes are at risk of exposure to airborne dusts.

Because their assigned protection factors are lower than those of other respirator types, the use of disposable or elastomeric half-facepiece respirators should be limited to situations where risks are low for inhaling material that might be contaminated with *H. capsulatum* spores. Situations that could be considered low risk include site surveys of bird roosts, collecting soil samples, or maintenance on filters of earthmoving equipment. However, during earthmoving activities at bird roosts or other work sites where the soil is known to be heavily contaminated by *H. capsulatum*, air-purifying, half-facepiece respirators should be worn by equipment operators to supplement dust suppression methods and the use of equipment with cabs.

Powered air-purifying respirators with loose-fitting facepiece and continuous-flow, supplied-air respirators with hood or helmet (assigned protection factor: 25)

A powered air-purifying respirator uses a small battery-operated blower to draw dusty air through attached filters and provides clean air at a constant flow rate of 170 liters per minute (L/min). This flow rate is usually greater than a wearer's breathing rate. Consequently, gaps in a face-to-facepiece seal will leak air outward rather than inward. Another advantage of these respirators is that they provide built-in eye protection. They are also the only respirators that adequately protect bearded workers.

Because powered air-purifying respirators cause almost no breathing resistance, the discomfort that some people experience while wearing a negative-pressure respirator is reduced. Interviews with 117 agricultural workers (53 swine farmers, 46 grain handlers, and 18 poultry farmers), found that powered air-purifying respirators with loose-fitting facepieces were rated best over disposable and elastomeric half-facepiece respirators for breathing ease, communication ease, skin comfort, and in-facepiece temperature and humidity.[119] Disposable respirators were rated best for weight and convenience.

Powered air-purifying respirators with particulate filters approved by NIOSH under the regulations of 42 CFR Part 84 have the prefix TC-84A. Only powered air-purifying respirators with high-efficiency filters are approved by NIOSH under Part 84.

Supplied-air respirators are not air-purifying types, but deliver breathing air from an air compressor or compressed air cylinder through a pressurized hose to the facepiece. Continuous-flow, supplied-air respirators with loose-fitting facepieces also provide a minimum air flow rate of 170 L/min. The maximum air flow rate of a continuous-flow supplied-air respirator may not exceed 425 L/min. Air supply hoses are available in a variety of lengths up to a maximum of 300 feet. All NIOSH-approved, supplied-air respirators have the prefix TC-19C.

An advantage of a supplied-air respirator is that the source of the breathing air does not depend upon filters to purify ambient air. An advantage of continuous-flow, supplied-air respirators is that when an activity involves work in a hot environment, such as an attic or a chicken house in the summer, a vortex tube can be added to the device that will cool the air flowing to the respirator wearer. A disadvantage of a supplied-air respirator is that if its air supply hose is too short, then mobility of the respirator wearer will be restricted. Also, in some situations (in attics or on elevated structures for example), the trailing hose of a supplied-air respirator can be a tripping hazard.

While the respirators described in this section have higher assigned protection factors than disposable or elastomeric half-facepiece respirators, they may not provide enough protection in extremely dusty conditions where air concentrations of *H. capsulatum* spores may be high, especially in enclosed spaces. Examples of activities for which respirators with higher assigned protection factors may be more important include cleaning chimneys[66] and working in attics[58,61,67] and poultry houses.[74–77]

Air-purifying, full-facepiece respirators; powered air-purifying respirators with half-facepiece or full facepiece; and continuous-flow, supplied-air respirators with half-facepiece or full facepiece (assigned protection factor: 50)

A full-facepiece respirator extends from the forehead to under the chin. It also has the built-in benefit of providing eye protection as well as respiratory

protection. As with other negative-pressure respirators, a complete face-to-facepiece seal is essential for good protection. However, partly because a good fit is easier with a full-facepiece, negative-pressure respirator, this type has a higher assigned protection factor than half-facepiece types. Fogging of a full-facepiece lens can obstruct vision, but this problem is preventable by adding a nosecup inside the facepiece. Antifogging agents in sticks and sprays are also available, but vary in their effectiveness. Most respirator manufacturers sell, but seldom advertise, packages of thin plastic covers for protecting the lens of a full-facepiece respirator. Available at a minimum charge, these replaceable covers prevent scratching of the permanent lens and prolong its life. NIOSH-approved, air-purifying, full-facepiece respirators for protection against particulate exposures have the prefix TC-84A.

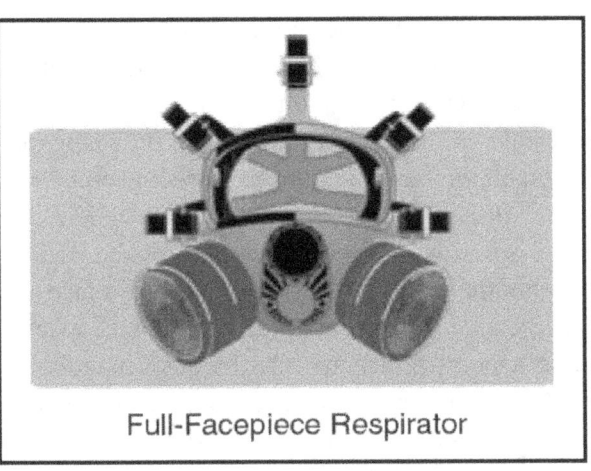

Full-Facepiece Respirator

The minimum air flow rate for both a powered air-purifying respirator and a continuous-flow, supplied-air respirator with a half-facepiece or full facepiece is 115 L/min. As with other continuous-flow, supplied-air respirators, the maximum air flow for these devices may not exceed 425 L/min. An air flow of 115 L/min is probably sufficient for most work activities involving possible exposures to aerosolized *H. capsulatum* spores. However, breathing rates during activities requiring heavy exertion may produce peak inhalation air flows exceeding 115 L/min. Consequently, someone doing heavy work could intermittently overbreathe the respirator's air flow, resulting in brief periods when contaminated air could enter the facepiece at gaps in the face-to-facepiece seal.

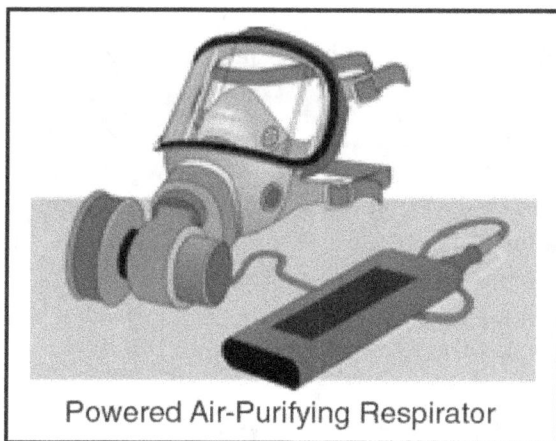

Powered Air-Purifying Respirator

The full-facepiece respirators described in this section are recommended as the minimum respiratory protection in extremely dusty conditions where high concentrations of *H. capsulatum* spores could be aerosolized, especially in enclosed areas. Air-purifying, full-facepiece respirators have been recommended for poultry workers based on the results of air sampling during chicken-catching activities inside poultry houses.[103] As mentioned earlier, half-facepiece respirators provide no eye protection, and even the concurrent use of eyecup goggles is probably impractical in extremely dusty working conditions. Unless the results of quantitative tests suggest that a person wearing an air-purifying, full-facepiece respirator can achieve an outstanding facepiece seal, a powered air-purifying respirator with a full facepiece should be chosen for extremely dusty work.

A powered air-purifying respirator with a full facepiece should also be the minimum respiratory protection worn by someone entering an enclosed area in which the amount of bat and bird manure contamination is unknown. A less protective respirator should be worn only when a site has been evaluated as having a low risk for inhalation exposure to material that might be contaminated with *H. capsulatum.*

Pressure-demand, supplied-air respirators with full facepiece (assigned protection factor: 2,000)

The air regulator of a pressure-demand, supplied-air respirator is designed to maintain positive facepiece pressure even during heavy physical activity. This type of respirator has the same advantages and disadvantages as other supplied-air respirators, except that a vortex tube cannot be used to cool the air delivered to the respirator wearer.

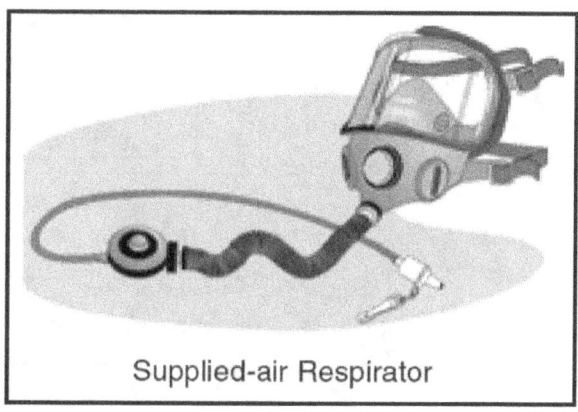

Supplied-air Respirator

Pressure-demand, self-contained breathing apparatuses (SCBA) and combination pressure-demand, supplied-air respirators with auxiliary SCBA (assigned protection factor: 10,000)

Because the wearer of a self-contained breathing apparatus (SCBA) carries his or her own air supply, a pressure-demand SCBA has an advantage of allowing greater mobility than a supplied-air respirator. However, not everyone may agree that this is a significant advantage, since these devices can weigh as much as 40 pounds. Open-circuit SCBAs, like those worn by firefighters, are available with rated service lives of 15, 30, 45, and 60 minutes. Auxiliary SCBAs for combination units are available that have service lives ranging from 3 to 60 minutes. Closed-circuit SCBAs, like those worn by members of mine rescue teams, are available with rated service lives from 1 to 4 hours.

SCBAs have been recommended for use by workers in areas contaminated with *H. capsulatum* spores,[100] but they are too impractical for most situations where respirators are needed to protect against the inhalation of *H. capsulatum* spores. Another disadvantage, particularly during removal jobs that may take a long time, is that SCBA can be used for only 30 to 60 minutes. Thus, frequent work stoppages are needed to change air cylinders. Also, an adequate supply of full cylinders is needed at a work site.

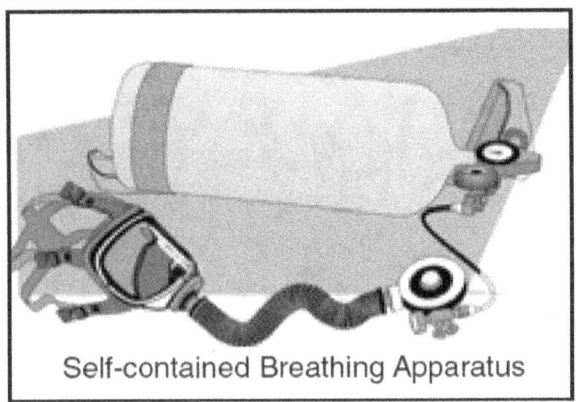

Self-contained Breathing Apparatus

Combination pressure-demand, supplied-air respirators with auxiliary SCBA would be useful for very dusty work environments. The auxiliary SCBA could be used to escape to an area of fresh air whenever delivery of breathing air is interrupted. All NIOSH-approved SCBA and combination SCBA and supplied-air respirators have the prefix TC-13F.

Summary

Because of the need for mobility, most decisions concerning the appropriate respirator for protecting against inhalation exposure to material that might contain *H. capsulatum* spores will involve choosing the most appropriate air-purifying respirator. To help the reader with this decision, Table 1 summarizes the advantages and disadvantages of air-purifying respirators and their costs.

What personal protective equipment other than respirators should workers wear?

Disposable protective clothing and shoe coverings should be worn whenever regular work clothing and shoes might be contaminated with dust containing *H. capsulatum* spores.[44,57,58] Wearing such clothing can reduce or eliminate the likelihood of transferring spore-contaminated dust to places away from a work site, such as a car or home. When spore-contaminated material is likely to fall from overhead, workers should wear disposable protective clothing with hoods.[58] Workers should wear disposable shoe coverings with ridged soles made of slip-resistant material to reduce the likelihood of slipping on wet or dusty surfaces. After working in a spore-contaminated area and before removing respirators, workers should remove all protective clothing and shoe coverings and seal them in heavy-duty plastic bags to be disposed of in a landfill.[120]

Since the personal protective equipment described above can be more insulating than regular work clothing, sweat evaporation may be impeded during some work activities. Therefore, precautions may need to be taken to control heat stress. For example, when protective clothing is needed, wearing a lightweight, cotton coverall would create less of a heat-stress risk for a worker than wearing a chemical-resistant suit. Additionally, workers should know the symptoms of heat-stress-related illnesses and be able to take appropriate measures to ensure that such illnesses do not occur. Some jobs may have such a significant risk of heat stress that they should be scheduled only when ambient temperatures are relatively cool.

Wearing chemical-resistant gloves will seldom be necessary when working in a spore-contaminated area. If they are worn, care should be taken to avoid the harmful effects on the skin that can result from occlusion (physical process of trapping a material against the skin), sweating, and maceration (softening and breaking down of tissue).[121,122] A thin cotton glove can be worn inside a chemical-resistant glove to protect against dermatitis, which can occur from prolonged skin exposure to moisture in gloves caused by perspiration. Because wearing chemical-resistant gloves can aggravate existing dermatitis, their use by workers having dermatitis may not be appropriate. The medical treatment of workers

Table 1. Air-Purifying Respirators

Respirator type	NIOSH assigned protection factor[106]	Advantages	Disadvantages	Cost (2004 dollars)
Filtering facepiece (Disposable)	10	– lightweight – no maintenance or cleaning needed – no effect on mobility	– provides no eye protection – can add to heat burden – inward leakage at gaps in face seal – some do not have adjustable head straps – difficult for a user to do a seal check – level of protection varies greatly among models – communication may be difficult – fit testing required to select proper facepiece size – some eyewear may interfere with the fit	$0.70 to $10
Elastomeric half-facepiece	10	– low maintenance – reusable facepiece and replaceable filters and cartridges – no effect on mobility	– provides no eye protection – can add to heat burden – inward leakage at gaps in face seal – communication may be difficult – fit testing required to select proper facepiece size – some eyewear may interfere with the fit	facepiece: $12 to $35 filters: $4 to $8 each
Powered with loose-fitting facepiece	25	– provides eye protection – protection for people with beards, missing dentures or facial scars – low breathing resistance – flowing air creates cooling effect – face seal leakage is generally outward – fit testing is not required – prescription glasses can be worn – communication less difficult than with elastomeric half-facepiece or full-facepiece respirators – reusable components and replaceable filters	– added weight of battery and blower – awkward for some tasks – battery requires charging – air flow must be tested with flow device before use	unit: $400 to $1000 filters: $10 to $30
Elastomeric full-facepiece with N-100, R-100, or P-100 filters	50	– provides eye protection – low maintenance – reusable facepiece and replaceable filters and cartridges – no effect on mobility – more effective face seal than that of filtering facepiece or elastomeric half-facepiece respirators	– can add to heat burden – diminished field-of-vision compared to half-facepiece – inward leakage at gaps in face seal – fit testing required to select proper facepiece size – facepiece lens can fog without nose cup or lens treatment – spectacle kit needed for people who wear corrective glasses	facepiece: $90 to $240 filters: $4 to $8 each nose cup: $30
Powered with tight-fitting half-facepiece or full-facepiece	50	– provides eye protection with full-facepiece – low breathing resistance – face seal leakage is generally outward – flowing air creates cooling effect – reusable components and replaceable filters	– added weight of battery and blower – awkward for some tasks – no eye protection with half-facepiece – fit testing required to select proper facepiece size – battery requires charging – communication may be difficult – spectacle kit needed for people who wear corrective glasses with full face-piece respirators – air flow must be tested with flow device before use	unit: $500 to $1000 filters: $10 to $30

Note: The assigned protection factors in this table are from the *NIOSH Respirator Selection Logic*.[106] When the table was prepared, OSHA had proposed amending the respiratory protection standard to incorporate assigned protection factors.[107] The Internet sites of NIOSH (www.cdc.gov/niosh) and OSHA (www.osha.gov) should be checked for the current assigned protection factor values.

having dermatitis and decisions about their use of gloves should be supervised by a physician experienced with occupational skin diseases.[122]

What other infectious agents are health risks for workers who disturb accumulations of bat droppings or bird manure?

In addition to *H. capsulatum*, inhalation exposure to *Cryptococcus neoformans* may also be a health risk for workers in environments containing accumulations of bat droppings or bird manure. Inhalation exposures to *Chlamydia psittaci* have occurred occasionally in environments containing the manure of certain birds, and exposure to the rabies virus is a health risk for workers who must handle dead bats.

Cryptococcus neoformans

C. neoformans is the infectious agent of the fungal disease cryptococcosis. Formerly a rare disease, the incidence of cryptococcosis has increased in recent years because of its frequent occurrence in AIDS patients.[123–127] *C. neoformans* and *H. capsulatum* are only two of the more than 100 microorganisms that have been reported with increased frequency among HIV-infected persons, and cryptococcosis and histoplasmosis are both classified as AIDS-indicator opportunistic infectious diseases.[127] In 1997, the USPHS/IDSA Prevention of Opportunistic Infections Working Group recommended that HIV-infected persons should avoid "sites that are likely to be heavily contaminated with *C. neoformans* (e.g., areas heavily contaminated with pigeon droppings)."[128] However, evidence is lacking that contaminated bird manure is the primary environmental source of exposure to *C. neoformans* in most cases of cryptococcosis among HIV-infected persons.[125] Thus, the 2001 USPHS/IDSA guidelines do not include the pigeon droppings example.[89] An HIV-infected person should consult his or her health care provider about the appropriate exposure precautions to be taken for any activity having a risk of exposure to *C. neoformans*.

C. neoformans uses the creatinine in avian feces as a nitrogen source. It gains a competitive advantage over other microorganisms and multiplies exceedingly well in dry bird manure accumulated in places that are not in direct sunlight.[38,123] This microorganism is commonly associated with old pigeon manure, but it has also been recovered from dried excreta of chickens, sparrows, starlings, and other birds.[123] As with *H. capsulatum*, *C. neoformans* has not been found in fresh bird droppings, but it has been cultured from the beaks and feet of pigeons.[123] Bats have been shown to be infected with *C. neoformans*,[129] and both *C. neoformans* and *H. capsulatum* have been recovered from bat dropping samples collected at the same site.[66,67] However, it should not be assumed that a worker's illness is cryptococcosis when only *C. neoformans* is recovered from environmental samples collected from suspected sources of exposure. *C. neoformans* has been recovered from environments where *H. capsulatum* was not recovered, even though sick workers were diagnosed from the results of clinical tests as having histoplasmosis.[61,86]

Unlike outbreaks of other mycoses, outbreaks of cryptococcosis traced to environmental sources have not been described, and it is presumed that most people can overcome most inhalation exposures to *C. neoformans*.[124] More detailed information about *C. neoformans* and cryptococcosis is available in other reports.[123,124,130–133] Work practices described previously in this document for controlling exposures to *H. capsulatum*, including the use of personal protective equipment, will also protect against inhalation exposures to *C. neoformans* and other microorganisms.

Chlamydia psittaci

Psittacosis is caused by a bacterium (*C. psittaci*) rather than a fungus, but it is another infectious disease that people can develop after disturbing and inhaling contaminated bird manure. While *C. psittaci* has been isolated from approximately 130 avian species,[134] most human infections result from inhalation exposures to aerosolized urine, respiratory secretions, or dried manure of infected psittacine (parrot-type) birds, such as cockatiels, parakeets, parrots, and macaws; avian chlamydiosis is diagnosed less frequently in canaries and finches.[135] Among caged, nonpsittacine birds, infection with *C. psittaci* occurs most frequently in pigeons, doves, mynah birds. Psittacosis in humans has occasionally been associated with exposures to infected pigeons, turkeys, chickens, ducks, pheasants, and geese, or their manure.[83,134,136–138]

According to the CDC's annual summaries of notifiable diseases, 904 cases of psittacosis in humans were reported to CDC from 1988 through 2003 (range: 15 cases in 2003 to 116 cases in 1989). Psittacosis is not a notifiable disease in all states, and thus, the actual number of cases is likely to be higher. Also, the number of cases may be underestimated because the disease is difficult to diagnose and cases often go unreported.[135] The severity of disease experienced by an infected person can range from asymptomatic to severe systemic disease with pneumonia; death occurs in less than 1% of properly treated patients.[135]

The National Association of State Public Health Veterinarians has recommended that workers should wear protective clothing, gloves, and a respirator with filters having an N-95 rating or higher when cleaning cages or handling birds infected with *C. psittaci*.[135]

Rabies

Rabies is a viral disease caused by infection of the central nervous systems of wild and domestic animals and humans.[139] The initial symptoms of human rabies resemble those of other systemic viral infections, including fever, headache, malaise, and disorders of the upper respiratory and gastrointestinal tracts.[140] Recognizing that a person has been exposed to the virus and prompt treatment are essential for preventing rabies. For once clinical symptoms have begun, there is no treatment for rabies and almost all patients will die from the disease or its complications within a few weeks of onset.[139,140]

In the United States, wild animals (especially bats, raccoons, skunks, coyotes, and foxes) are the most important sources of rabies infection.[141–143] Indigenous rabid bats have been reported from every state except Hawaii.[141–143] Individual bats from most of the estimated 41 bat species in the United States have been found to be infected with rabies virus.[145] Rabies virus associated with insectivorous bats (those that feed principally on insects) accounted for 32 of the 35 indigenous rabies cases in humans in the United States between 1958 and 2000.[145]

Rabies is transmitted via an infected animal's bite or by contamination of abrasions, open wounds, mucous membranes or theoretically, scratches, by infectious material such as saliva.[144] Contact with the blood, urine, or manure of a rabid animal is not a risk factor for contracting rabies.[144] Consequently, workers exposed to accumulations of bat droppings in environments from which bats have been excluded have no rabies risk. Although spelunkers seldom have direct contact with bats, they are included in a frequent-risk category by CDC because of potential for bite, nonbite, or aerosol exposure to the rabies virus.[144] Two fatal cases of rabies in humans have been attributed to possible airborne exposures in caves containing millions of free-tailed bats.[144] In addition, between 1990 and 2000, a bite was documented in only 2 of the 24 U.S. human rabies cases caused by bat-associated rabies virus variants.[146] This suggests "that transmission of rabies virus can occur from minor, seemingly unimportant, or unrecognized bites from bats."[144] While aerosol transmission of the rabies virus from bats to people is theoretically possible under extraordinary conditions, the risk is otherwise negligible.

The percentage of rabid bats in any colony is probably low (0.5% or less[95]). However, a dead bat should still never be picked up with bare hands since its death may have been caused by an infectious agent. The rabies virus can remain infectious in a carcass until decomposition is well advanced.[94] Thus, whenever possible, a shovel or some other tool should be used to pick up and dispose of a dead bat. If a dead bat must be handled, wearing heavy work gloves should minimize the risk of disease transmission because of an accidental scratch from the bat's teeth or by contamination of existing scratches or abrasions on a worker's hands.

Where can I get more information about infectious diseases and answers to questions about worker health and safety issues?

This guidance document was prepared by the National Institute for Occupational Safety and Health (NIOSH) and the National Center for Infectious Diseases (NCID), both of the Centers for Disease Control and Prevention. For more information about histoplasmosis or other infectious diseases, please contact your physician, your local health department, or NCID in Atlanta, Georgia, NCID's Internet address is http://www.cdc.gov/ncidod/. For more information about worker health and safety precautions during disturbances of soil, bat droppings, or bird manure that might be contaminated with *H. capsulatum spores*, call NIOSH in Cincinnati, Ohio, at (800) 356-4674. A list of non-powered, air-purifying respirators that have been tested and approved by NIOSH under 42 CFR Part 84 regulations can be found on the NIOSH Internet home page, http://www.cdc.gov/niosh.

References

1. Heymann DL, ed. [2004]. Control of communicable diseases manual. 18th ed. Washington, DC: American Public Health Association, pp. 273–275.

2. Walsh TJ, Larone DH, Schell WA, Mitchell TG [2003]. Chapter 118: *Histoplasma, Blastomyces, Coccidioides*, and other dimorphic fungi causing systemic mycoses. In: Murray PR, editor-in-chief. Manual of clinical microbiology. 8th ed. Washington, DC: American Society for Microbiology Press, pp. 1781–1797.

3. Deepe GS Jr. [2000]. Chapter 254: *Histoplasma capsulatum*. In: Mandell GL, Bennett JE, Dolin R, eds. Principles and practices of infectious diseases. 5th ed. Philadelphia, PA: Churchill Livingstone, pp. 2718–2733.

4. Cano MVC, Hajjeh RA [2001]. The epidemiology of histoplasmosis: a review. Semin. Respir. Infect. 16(2):109–118.

5. Wheat LJ [2000]. Chapter 3: Histoplasmosis. In: Sarosi GA, Davies SF, eds. Fungal Diseases of the Lung. 3rd ed. Philadelphia, PA: Lippincott Williams and Wilkins, pp. 31–46.

6. Johnson PC, Sarosi GA [1987]. Histoplasmosis. Semin. Respir. Med. 9(2):145–151.

7. Larsh HW [1983]. Histoplasmosis. In: DiSalvo AF, ed. Occupational mycoses. Philadelphia, PA: Lea and Febiger, pp. 29–41.

8. Mitchell TG [1992]. Systemic mycoses. In: Joklik WK, Willett HP, Amos DB, Wifert CM, eds. Zinsser microbiology. 20th ed. Norwalk, CT: Appleton and Lange, pp. 1091–1112.

9. Furcolow ML, Schubert J, Tosh FE, Doto IL, Lynch HJ Jr. [1962]. Serologic evidence of histoplasmosis in sanatoriums in the US. JAMA 180:109–114.

10. Wheat LJ, Kauffman CA [2003]. Histoplasmosis. Fungal infections, part II: recent advances in diagnosis, treatment, and prevention of endemic and cutaneous mycoses. Infect. Dis. Clin. N. Am. 17:1–19.

11. Wheat J, Sarosi G, McKinsey D, Hamill R, Bradsher R, Johnson P, Loyd J, Kauffman C [2000]. Practice guidelines for the management of patients with histoplasmosis. Clin. Infect. Dis. 30:688–695.

12. Wheat LJ, Connolly-Stringfield PA, Baker RL, Curfman MF, Eads ME, Israel KS, Norris SA, Webb DH, Zeckel ML [1990]. Disseminated histoplasmosis in the acquired immune deficiency syndrome: clinical findings, diagnosis and treatment, and review of the literature. Med. 69(6):361–374.

13. Deepe GS [1994]. The immune response to *Histoplasma capsulatum*: unearthing its secrets. J. Lab. Clin. Med. 123:201–205.

14. Davies SF [1990]. Histoplasmosis: update 1989. Semin. Respir. Infections 5 (2):93–104.

15. Hajjeh RA [1995]. Disseminated histoplasmosis in persons infected with human immunodeficiency virus. Clin. Infectious Dis. 21 (Suppl 1):S108–S110.

16. Wheat LJ, Slama TG, Zeckel ML [1985]. Histoplasmosis in the acquired immune deficiency syndrome. Am. J. Med. 78:203–210.

17. Greenfield RA [1989]. Pulmonary infections due to higher bacteria and fungi in the immuno compromised host. Semin. Respir. Med. 10:68–77.

18. Selik RM, Karon JM, Ward JW [1997]. Effect of the human immunodeficiency virus epidemic on mortality from opportunistic infections in the United States in 1993. J. Infect. Dis. 176:632–636.

19. Deepe GS Jr. [1997]. *Histoplasma capsulatum*: Darling of the river valleys. ASM News 63:599–604.

20. Ciulla TA [undated]. Presumed ocular histoplasmosis syndrome. Available from the Web site of MiraVisa Diagnostics. [http://www.miravistalabs.com/refLibrary_reviews_page.php?id=40]. Date accessed: September 2004.

21. National Eye Institute [2004]. Histoplasmosis. [http://www.nei.nih.gov/health/histoplasmosis/index.asp]. Date accessed: September 2004.

22. Schwarz J [1981]. Histoplasmosis of the eye. In: Histoplasmosis. New York, NY: Praeger Publishers, pp. 317–350.

23. Newell FW [1992]. Ophthalmology principles and concepts. 7th ed. St. Louis, MO: Mosby Year Book, p. 439.

24. Daniel TM, Baum GL [2002]. Drama and discovery, the story of histoplasmosis. Westport, CN: Greenwood Press, p. 109.

25. Wheat LJ [1992]. Histoplasmosis in Indianapolis. Clin. Infectious Dis. 14 (Suppl 1):S91–S99.

26. Wheat J, French MLV, Kohler RB, Zimmerman SE, Smith CD, Slama TG [1982]. The diagnostic laboratory tests for histoplasmosis. Ann. Int. Med. 97(5):680–685.

27. George RB, Penn RL [1986]. Histoplasmosis. In: Sarosi GA, Davies SF, eds. Fungal diseases of the lung. Orlando, FL: Harcourt Brace Jovanovich, pp. 69–85.

28. Bracca A, Tosello ME, Girardini JE, Amigot SL, Gomez C, Serra E [2003]. Molecular detection of *Histoplasma capsulatum* var. *capsulatum* in human clinical samples. J. Clin. Microbiol. 41:1753–1755.

29. Guedes HL, Guimarães AJ, Muniz M, Pizzini VC, Hamilton AJ, Peralta JM, Deepe GS Jr, Zancopé-Oliveira RM [2003]. PCR assay for identification of *Histoplasma capsulatum* based on the nucleotide sequence of the M antigen. J. Clin. Microbiol. 41:535–539.

30. Rickerts V, Bialek R, Tintelnot K, Jacobi V, Just-Nübling G [2002]. Rapid PCR-based diagnosis of disseminated histoplasmosis in an AIDS patient. Eur. J. Clin. Infect. Dis. *21*:821–823.

31. Reiss E, Kaufman L, Kovacs JA, Lindsley MD [2002]. Chapter 61: Clinical immunomycology. In: Rose NR, Hamilton RG, Detrick B, eds. Manual of clinical laboratory immunology. 6th ed. Washington, DC: American Society for Microbiology Press, pp. 559–583.

32. Sutton DA [2003]. Chapter 111: Specimen collection, transport, and processing: mycology. In: Murray PR, Baron EJ, Jorgensen JH, Pfaller MA, Yolken RH, eds. Manual of clinical microbiology. 8th ed. Washington, DC: American Society for Microbiology Press, pp. 1659–1667.

33. Richmond RY, McKinney RW, eds. [1999]. Biosafety in microbiological and biomedical laboratories. 4th ed. [http://www.cdc.gov/od/ohs/biosfty/bmbl4/bmbl4toc.htm]. Date accessed: September 2004.

34. Rippon JW [1988]. Chapter 15: Histoplasmosis (histoplasmosis capsulati and histoplasmosis farciminosum).In: Medical mycology: the pathogenic fungi and the pathogenic actinomycetes.3rd ed. Philadelphia, PA: W.B. Saunders Company, pp. 381–423.

35. Wheat LJ, Kohler RB, Tewari RP:[1986]. Diagnosis of disseminated histoplasmosis by detection of *Histoplasma capsulatum* antigen in serum and urine specimens. N. Engl. J. Med. *314*:83–88.

36. Wheat LJ, Connolly-Stringfield P, Kohler RB, Frame PT, Gupta MR [1989]. *Histoplasma capsulatum* polysaccharide antigen detection in diagnosis and management of disseminated histoplasmosis in patients with acquired immunodeficiency syndrome. Am. J. Med. *87*:396–400.

37. Edwards LB, Acquaviva FA, Livesay VT [1973]. Further observations on histoplasmin sensitivity in the United States. Am. J. Epidemiol. *98*(5):315–325.

38. Ajello L, Weeks RJ [1983]. Soil decontamination and other control measures. In: DiSalvo AF, ed. Occupational mycoses. Philadelphia, PA: Lea and Febiger, pp. 229–238.

39. Stobierski MG, Hospedales CJ, Hall WN, Robinson-Dunn B, Hoch D, Sheill DA [1996]. Outbreak of histoplasmosis among employees in a paper factory—Michigan, 1993. J. Clin. Microbiol. *34*(5):1220–1223.

40. Morse DL, Gordon MA, Matte T, Eadie G [1985]. An outbreak of histoplasmosis in a prison. Am. J. Epidemiol. *122*(2):253–261.

41. Bartlett PC, Weeks RJ, Ajello L [1982]. Decontamination of *Histoplasma capsulatum*-infested bird roost in Illinois. Arch. Environ. Health *37*:221–223.

42. Gustafson TL, Kaufman L, Weeks R, Ajello L, Hutcheson RH, Wiener SL, et al. [1981]. Outbreak of acute pulmonary histoplasmosis in members of a wagon train. Am. J. Med. *71*:759–765.

43. Chick EW, Compton SB, Pass III T, Mackey B, Hernandez C, Austin Jr E, et al. [1981]. Hitchcock's birds, or the increased rate of exposure to Histoplasma from blackbird roost sites. Chest *80*(4):434–438.

44. Storch G, Burford JG, George RB, Kaufman L, Ajello L [1980]. Acute histoplasmosis. Description of an outbreak in northern Louisiana. Chest *77*:38–42.

45. DiSalvo AF, Johnson WM [1979]. Histoplasmosis in South Carolina: support for the microfocus concept. Am. J. Epidemiol. *109*(4):480–492.

46. Latham RH, Kaiser AB, Dupont WD, Dan BB [1980]. Chronic pulmonary histoplasmosis following the excavation of a bird roost. Am. J. Med. *68*:504–508.

47. Sarosi GA, Parker JD, Tosh FE [1971]. Histoplasmosis outbreaks: their patterns. In: Ajello L, Chick EW, Furcolow ML, eds. Histoplasmosis: proceedings of the second national conference. Springfield, IL: Charles C. Thomas, pp. 123–128.

48. Tosh FE, Weeks RJ, Pfeiffer FR, Hendricks SL, Greer DL, Chin TDY [1967]. The use of formalin to kill *Histoplasma capsulatum* at an epidemic site. Am. J. Epidemiol. *85*:259–265.

49. Tosh FE, Weeks RJ, Pfeiffer FR, Hendricks SL, Chin TDY [1966]. Chemical decontamination of soil containing *Histoplasma capsulatum*. Am. J. Epidemiol. *83*:262–270.

50. Tosh FE, Doto IL, D'Alessio DJ, Medeiros AA, Hendricks SL, Chin TDY [1966]. The second of two epidemics of histoplasmosis resulting from work on the same starling roost. Am. Rev. Respir. Dis. *94*:406–413.

51. Weeks RJ [1984]. Histoplasmosis sources of infection and methods of control. Atlanta, GA: Centers for Disease Control and Prevention.

52. Dean AG, Bates JH, Sorrels C, Sorrels T, Germany W, Ajello L, Kaufman L, McGrew C, Fitts A [1978]. An outbreak of histoplasmosis at an Arkansas courthouse, with five cases of probable reinfection. Am. J. Epidemiol. *108*:36–46.

53. Raphael SS, Schwarz J [1953]. Occupational hazards from fungi causing deep mycoses. Arch. Ind. Hyg. Occup. Med. *8*:154–165.

54. Felson B, Jones GF, Ulrich RP [1950]. Roentgenologic aspects of diffuse miliary granulomatous pneumonitis of unknown etiology: report of twelve cases with eighteen months' follow-up. Am. J. Roentgenol. Radium Ther. *64*(5):740–746.

55. Jones TF, Swinger GL, Craig AS, McNeil MM, Kaufman L, Schaffner W [1999]. Acute pulmonary histoplasmosis in bridge workers: a persistent problem. Am. J. Med. *106*:480–482.

56. Valdez H, Salata RA [1999]. Bat-associated histoplasmosis in returning travelers: case presentation and description of a cluster. J. Travel Med. *6*:258–260.

57. Leslie L, Arnette C, Sikder A, Adams J, Holbrook C, Bond J, King B, Roberts K, Patrick MS, Palmer C, Finger R, Tomford JW, Rushton T [1995]. Histoplasmosis—Kentucky, 1995. MMWR *44*(38):701–703.

58. Lenhart SW [1994]. Recommendations for protecting workers from *Histoplasma capsulatum* exposure during bat guano removal from a church's attic. Appl. Occup. Environ. Hyg. *9*:230–236.

59. Gordon SM, Reines SS, Alvarado CS, Nolte F, Keyserling HL, Bryan J [1993]. Disseminated histoplasmosis caused by *Histoplasma capsulatum* in an immuno compromised adolescent after exploration of a bat cave. Pediatric Infect. Dis. J. *12*(1):102–104.

60. Sacks JJ, Ajello L, Crockett LK [1986]. An outbreak and review of cave-associated histoplasmosis capsulati. J. Med. Vet. Mycol. *24*:313–325.

61. Bartlett PC, Vonbehren LA, Tewari RP, Martin RJ, Eagleton L, Isaac MJ, Kulkarni PS [1982]. Bats in the belfry: an outbreak of histoplasmosis. Am. J. Public Health *72*:1369–1372.

62. Schwarz J [1981]. Bats and soil. In: Histoplasmosis. New York, NY: Praeger Publishers, pp. 179–186.

63. Sorley DL, Levin ML, Warren JW, Flynn JPG, Gerstenblith J [1979]. Bat-associated histoplasmosis in Maryland bridge workers. Am. J. Med. *67*:623–626.

64. Chick EW, Bauman DS, Lapp NL, Morgan WKC [1972]. A combined field and laboratory epidemic of histoplasmosis. Am. Rev. Respir. Dis. *105*:968–971.

65. DiSalvo AF [1971]. The role of bats in the ecology of *Histoplasma capsulatum*. In: Ajello L, Chick EW, Furcolow ML, eds. Histoplasmosis: proceedings of the second national conference. Springfield, IL: Charles C. Thomas, pp. 149–161.

66. Gordon MA, Ziment I [1967]. Epidemic of acute histoplasmosis in western New York State. N.Y. State J. Med. *67*:235–243.

67. Ajello L, Hosty TS, Palmer J [1967]. Bat histoplasmosis in Alabama. Am. J. Trop. Med. Hyg. *16*:329–331.

68. Hasenclever HF, Shacklette MH, Young RV, Gelderman GA [1967]. The natural occurrence of *Histoplasma capsulatum* in a cave—1. Epidemiologic aspects. Am. J. Epidemiol. *86*(1):238–245.

69. Shacklette MH, Hasenclever HF, Miranda EA [1967]. The natural occurrence of *Histoplasma capsulatum* in a cave—2. Ecologic aspects. Am. J. Epidemiol. *86*(1):246–252.

70. Shacklette MH, Hasenclever HF [1967]. The natural occurrence of *Histoplasma capsulatum* in a cave—3. Effect of flooding. Am. J. Epidemiol. *88*(2):210–252.

71. Campins H, Zubillaga C, Lopez LG, Dorante M [1956]. An epidemic of histoplasmosis in Venezuela. Am. J. Trop. Med. *5*:690–695.

72. Englert E, Phillips AW [1953]. Acute diffuse pulmonary granulomatosis in bridge workers. Am. J. Med. *15*:733–740.

73. Scalia SP [1961]. An outbreak of histoplasmosis in Baltimore County. Maryland State Med. J. *10*:614–619.

74. Lehan PH, Furcolow ML [1957]. Epidemic histoplasmo sis. J. Chron. Dis. *5*(4):489–503.

75. Furcolow ML, Menges RW, Larsh HW [1955]. An epidemic of histoplasmosis involving man and animals. Ann. Int. Med. *43*:173–181.

76. Imbach MJ, Larsh HW, Furcolow ML [1954]. Epidemic histoplasmosis and airborne *Histoplasma capsulatum*. Proc. Soc. Exper. Biol. and Med. *85*:72–74.

77. Zeidberg LD, Ajello L [1954]. Environmental factors influencing the occurrence of *Histoplasma capsulatum* and *Microsporum gypseum* in soil. J. Bacteriol. *68*:156–159.

78. Kier JH, Campbell CC, Ajello L, Sutliff WD [1954]. Acute bronchopneumonic histoplasmosis following exposure to infected garden soil. J. Am. Med. Assoc. *155*:1230–1232.

79. Schwarz J [1981]. Global epidemiology and distribution of histoplasmosis. In: Histoplasmosis. New York, NY: Praeger Publishers, p. 87.

80. Hasenclever HF [1979]. Impact of airborne pathogens in outdoor systems: histoplasmosis. In: Edmonds RL, ed. Aerobiology: the ecological systems approach. Stroudsburg, PA: Dowden, Hutchinson and Ross, Inc., pp. 199–208.

81. Kassa H, Harrington B, Bisesi MS [2001]. Risk of occupational exposure to *Cryptosporidium*, *Giardia*, and *Campylobacter* associated with the feces of giant Canada Geese. Appl. Occup. Environ. Hyg. *16*:905–909.

82. Feare CJ, Sanders MF, Blasco R, Bishop JD [1999]. Canada goose (*Branta canadensis*) droppings as a potential source of pathogenic bacteria. J. Royal Soc. Promot. Health *119*:146–155.

83. Converse K, Wolcott M, Docherty D, Cole R, [1999]. Screening for potential human pathogens in fecal material deposited by resident Canada geese on areas of public utility. Available from the Web site of the National Wildlife Health Center. [http://www.nwhc.usgs.gov/pub_metadata/canada_geese.html]. Date accessed: September 2004.

84. Ward JI, Weeks M, Allen M, Hutcheson RH Jr., Anderson R, Fraser DW et al. [1979]. Acute histoplasmosis: clinical, epidemiologic and serologic findings of an outbreak associated with exposure to a fallen tree. Am. J. Med. *66*:587–595.

85. Schlech WF, Wheat LJ, Ho JL, French MLV, Weeks RJ, Kohler RB, Deane CE, Eitzen HE, Band JD [1983]. Recurrent urban histoplasmosis, Indianapolis, Indiana, 1980–1981. Am. J. Epidemiol. *118*:301–312.

86. Schwarz J, Kauffman CA [1977]. Occupational hazards from deep mycoses. Arch. Dermatol. *113*:1270–1275.

87. Reid TM, Schafer MP [1999]. Direct detection of *Histoplasma capsulatum* in soil suspensions by two-stage PCR. Mol. Cell. Probes *13*:269–273.

88. Wheat LJ, Slama TG, Norton JA, Kohler RB, Eitzen HE, French MLV, Sathapatayavongs B [1982]. Risk factors for disseminated or fatal histoplasmosis, analysis of a large urban outbreak. Ann. Intern. Med. *96*:159–163.

89. U.S. Public Health Service (USPHS) and Infectious Diseases Society of America (IDSA) [2001]. 2001 USPHS/IDSA guidelines for the prevention of opportunistic infections in persons infected with human immunodeficiency virus. [http://www.aidsinfo.nih.gov/guidelines/op_infections/O-I_112801.pdf]. Date accessed: September 2004.

90. Wilcox KR Jr., Waisbren BA, Martin J [1958]. The Walworth, Wisconsin, epidemic of histoplasmosis. Ann. Intern. Med. *49*:388–418.

91. Byrd RB, Leavey R, Trunk G [1975]. The Chanute histoplasmosis epidemic. Chest *68*(6):791–795.

92. Brodsky AL, Gregg MB, Loewenstein MS, Kaufman L, Mallison GF [1973]. Outbreak of histoplasmosis associated with the 1970 earth day activities. Am. J. Med. *54*:333–342.

93. Chamany S, Mirza S, Fleming J, Howell, Lenhart SW, Mortimer VD, et al. [2004]. A large histoplasmosis outbreak among high school students in Indiana, 2001. Pediatr. Infect. Dis. J. *23*(10):909–914.

94. Greenhall AM, Frantz SC [1994]. Bats In: Prevention and control of wildlife damage. [http://www.ces.ncsu.edu/nreos/wild/wildlife/wdc/]. Date accessed: September 2004.

95. Tuttle MD [1988]. America's neighborhood bats. Austin, TX: University of Texas Press.

96. Bat Conservation International, Inc. [1996]. Exclusion experts promote pest control industry changes. Bats *14*(2):10–11.

97. Williams DE, Corrigan RM [1994]. Pigeons (rock doves). In: Prevention and control of wildlife damage. [http://www.ces.ncsu.edu/nreos/wild/wildlife/wdc/]. Date accessed: September 2004.

98. Agency for Toxic Substances and Disease Registry [1999]. Toxicological profile for formaldehyde. Atlanta, GA: U.S. Department of Health and Human Services, Public Health Service. [http://www.atsdr.cdc.gov/toxprofiles/tp111.pdf]. Date accessed: September 2004.

99. Smith CD, Furcolow ML, Tosh FE [1964]. Attempts to eliminate *Histoplasma capsulatum* from soil. Am. J. Hyg. *79*(2):170–180.

100. CDC [1977]. Histoplasmosis control: decontamination of bird roosts, chicken houses and other point sources. Atlanta, GA: Centers for Disease Control and Prevention.

101. Wheat J [1997]. Histoplasmosis: experience during outbreaks in Indianapolis and review of the literature. Med. *76*:339–354.

102. USDA, National Agricultural Statistics Service [2004]. Table 27. Poultry—inventory and number sold: 2002 and 1997. In: 2002 Census of Agriculture, Chapter 1. United States data.

103. Lenhart SW, Morris PD, Akin RE, Olenchock SA, Service WS, Boone WP [1990]. Organic dust, endotoxin, and ammonia exposures in the North Carolina poultry processing industry. Appl. Occup. Environ. Hyg. *5*(9):611–618.

104. Furcolow ML [1965]. Environmental aspects of histoplasmosis. Arch. Environ. Health *10*:4–10.

105. Myers WR, Lenhart SW, Campbell D, Provost G [1983]. Letter to the editor; topic: respirator performance terminology. Am. Ind. Hyg. Assoc. J. *44*(3):B25–B26.

106. NIOSH [2004]. NIOSH respirator selection logic. Cincinnati, OH: U.S. Department of Health and Human Services, Centers for Disease Control and Prevention, National Institute for Occupational Safety and Health, DHHS (NIOSH) Pub. No. 2005–100.

107. Occupational Safety and Health Administration. [2003]. Assigned protection factors; proposed rule. Federal Register *68*(109):34114.

108. American National Standards Institute. [1992]. American national standard for respiratory protection (ANSI Z88.2-1992). New York, NY: American National Standards Institute.

109. Lenhart SW, Seitz T, Trout D, Bollinger N [2004]. Issues affecting respirator selection for workers exposed to infectious aerosols: emphasis on healthcare settings. Applied Biosafety *9*:20–36.

110. Furcolow ML [1961]. Airborne histoplasmosis. Bacteriological Rev. *25*:301–309.

111. Imbach MJ, Larsh HW, Furcolow ML [1954]. Isolation of *Histoplasma capsulatum* from the air. Science *119*:71.

112. NIOSH [1987]. NIOSH guide to industrial respiratory protection. Cincinnati, OH: U.S. Department of Health and Human Services, Public Health Service, Centers for Disease Control, National Institute for Occupational Safety and Health, DHHS (NIOSH) Publication No. 87-116.

113. 63 Fed. Reg. 1152–1300 1998]. Occupational Safety and Health Administration: Respiratory protection; final rule. (Codified at 29 CFR Part 1910.134).

114. Oestenstad RK, Dillion HK, Perkins LL [1990]. Distribution of faceseal leak sites on a half-mask respirator and their association with facial dimensions. Am. Ind. Hyg. Assoc. J. 51:285–290.

115. 60 Fed. Reg. 30336 [1995]. National Institute for Occupational Safety and Health: Respiratory protective devices; final rule. (Codified at 42 CFR Part 84).

116. Campbell DL, Coffey CC, Lenhart SW [2001]. Respiratory protection as a function of respirator fitting characteristics and fit-test accuracy. Am. Ind. Hyg. Assoc. J. *62*:36–44.

117. Coffey CC, Lawrence RB, Campbell DL, Zhuang Z, Calvert CA, Jensen PA [2004]. Fitting characteristics of eighteen N95 filtering-facepiece respirators. J. Occup. Environ. Hyg. *1*:262–271.

118. Rey P, Meyer J-J [1998]. Vision and work. In: Stellman JM, ed. Encyclopaedia of Occupational Health and Safety. 4th ed. Geneva, Switzerland: International Labour Office, pp. 11.10–11.22.

119. Popendorf W, Merchant JA, Leonard S, Burmeister LF, Olenchock SA [1995]. Respirator protection and acceptability among agricultural workers. Appl. Occup. Environ. Hyg. *10*(7):595–605.

120. USAEHA [1992]. Managing health hazards associated with bird and bat excrement. Aberdeen Proving Ground, MD: U. S. Army Environmental Hygiene Agency, U. S. Army Environmental Hygiene Agency Technical Guide 142.

121. Wigger-Alberti W, Elsner P [1998]. Do barrier creams and gloves prevent or provoke contact dermatitis? Am. J. Contact Dermatitis *9*(2):100–106.

122. Mathias CGT [1990]. Prevention of occupational contact dermatitis. J. Am. Acad. Dermatol. *23*:742–748.

123. Hajjeh RA, Brandt ME, Pinner RW [1995]. Emergence of cryptococcal disease: epidemiologic perspectives 100 years after its discovery. Epidemiol. Rev. *17*(2):303–320.

124. Levitz SM [1991]. The ecology of *Cryptococcus neoformans* and the epidemiology of cryptococcosis. Rev. Infect. Dis. *13*:1163–1169.

125. Pinner RW, Hajjeh RA, Powderly WG [1995]. Prospects for preventing cryptococcosis in persons infected with human immunodeficiency virus. Clin. Infect. Dis. 21 (Suppl 1):S103– S107.

126. Mitchell TJ, Perfect JR [1995]. Cryptococcosis in the era of AIDS—100 years after the discovery of Cryptococcus neoformans. Clin. Microbiol. Rev. *8*:515–548.

127. Kaplan JE, Masur H, Holmes KK, McNeil MM, Schonberger LB, Navin TR, et al. [1995]. USPHS/IDSA guidelines for the prevention of opportunistic infections in persons infected with human immunodeficiency virus: introduction. Clin. Infect. Dis. *21* (suppl 1):S1–S11.

128. Centers for Disease Control and Prevention (CDC) [1997]. 1997 USPHS/IDSA guidelines for the prevention of opportunistic infections in persons infected with human immunodeficiency virus. MMWR 46 (No. RR-12):1–46.

129. Grose E, Marinkelle CJ, Striegel C [1968]. The use of tissue cultures in the identification of Cryptococcus neoformans isolated from Colombian bats. Sabouraudia *6*:127–132.

130. Mitchell TG [1992]. Opportunistic mycoses. In: Joklik WK, Willett HP, Amos DB, Wifert CM, eds. Zinsser microbiology. 20th ed. Norwalk, CT: Appleton and Lange, pp. 1135–1157.

131. Ehrensing ER, Saag MS [2000]. Chapter 7: Cryptococcosis. In: Sarosi GA, Davies SF, eds. Fungal diseases of the lung. 3rd ed. Orlando, FL: Lippincott Williams and Wilkins, pp. 91–103.

132. Diamond RD [2000]. Chapter 253: *Cryptococcus neoformans*. In: Mandell GL, Bennett JE, Dolin R, eds. Principles and practices of infectious diseases. 5th ed. Philadelphia, PA: Churchill Livingstone, pp. 2707–2718.

133. Buchanan KL, Murphy JW [1998]. What makes *Cryptococcus neoformans* a pathogen? Emerg. Infect. Dis. *4*:71–83.

134. Schlossberg D [2000]. Chapter 169: *Chlamydia psittaci* (Psittacosis). In: Mandell GL, Bennett JE, Dolin R, eds. Principles and practices of infectious diseases. 5th ed. Philadelphia, PA: Churchill Livingstone, pp. 2004–2007.

135. Centers for Disease Control and Prevention (CDC) [2000]. Compendium of measures to control *Chlamydia psittaci* infection among humans (psittacosis) and pet birds (avian chlamydiosis), 2000 and Compendium of animal rabies prevention and control, 2000: National Association of State Public Health Veterinarians, Inc. MMWR *49* (No. RR-8):1–17.

136. Heymann DL, ed. [2004]. Control of communicable diseases manual. 18th ed. Washington, DC: American Public Health Association, pp. 432–434.

137. Wyrick PB, Gutman LT, Hodinka RL [1992]. Chlamydiae. In: Joklik WK, Willett HP, Amos DB, Wifert CM, eds. Zinsser microbiology. 20th ed. Norwalk, CT: Appleton and Lange, pp. 719–729.

138. Centers for Disease Control and Prevention (CDC) [1990]. Psittaccosis at a turkey processing plant—North Carolina, 1989. MMWR *39*(27):460–469.

139. Hooper DC [2002]. Rabies virus. In: Rose NR, Hamilton RG, Detrick B, eds. Manual of clinical laboratory immunology. 6th ed. Washington, DC: American Society for Microbiology Press, pp. 742–748.

140. Bleck TP, Rupprecht CE [2000]. Chapter 151: Rabies virus. In: Mandell GL, Bennett JE, Dolin R, eds. Principles and practices of infectious diseases. 5th ed. Philadelphia, PA: Churchill Livingstone, pp. 1811–1820.

141. Centers for Disease Control and Prevention (CDC) [2000]. Compendium of measures to control *Chlamydia psittaci* infection among humans (psittacosis) and pet birds (avian chlamydiosis), 2000 and Compendium of animal rabies prevention and control, 2000: National Association of State Public Health Veterinarians, Inc. MMWR *49* (No. RR-8):19–30.

142. Centers for Disease Control and Prevention (CDC) [2004]. Compendium of animal rabies prevention and control, 2004: National Association of State Public Health Veterinarians, Inc. MMWR *53* (No. RR-9):1–6.

143. Rupprecht CE, Smith JS, Krebs J, Niezgoda M, Childs JE [1996]. Current issues in rabies prevention in the United States: health dilemmas, public coffers, private interests. Public Health Rep. *111*:400–407.

144. Centers for Disease control and Prevention [1999]. Human rabies prevention – United States, 1999: recommendations of the Advisory Committee on Immunization Practices (ACIP). MMWR *48* (No. RR-1):1–21.

145. Messenger SL, Smith JS, Rupprecht CE [2002]. Emerging epidemiology of bat-associated cryptic cases of rabies in humans in the United States. Clin. Infect. Dis. *35*:738–747.

146. Centers for Disease Control and Prevention (CDC) [2004]. Human death associated with bat rabies—California, 2003. MMWR *53*:33–35.

Appendix

HISTOPLASMOSIS

What is histoplasmosis?

Histoplasmosis is an infectious disease caused by inhaling spores of a fungus called *Histoplasma capsulatum*. Histoplasmosis is not contagious; it cannot be transmitted from an infected person or animal to someone else.

What are the symptoms of histoplasmosis?

Histoplasmosis primarily affects a person's lungs, and its symptoms vary greatly. The vast majority of infected people are asymptomatic (have no apparent ill effects) or they experience symptoms so mild they do not seek medical attention. If symptoms do occur, they will usually start within 3 to 17 days after exposure, with an average of 10 days. Histoplasmosis can appear as a mild, flu-like respiratory illness and has a combination of symptoms, including malaise (a general ill feeling), fever, chest pain, dry or nonproductive cough, headache, loss of appetite, shortness of breath, joint and muscle pains, chills, and hoarseness. A chest X-ray of a person with acute pulmonary histoplamosis will commonly show a patchy pneumonitis, which eventually calcifies. Chronic lung disease due to histoplasmosis resembles tuberculosis and can worsen over months or years. The most severe and rare form of this disease is disseminated histoplasmosis, which involves spreading of the fungus to other organs outside the lungs.

Who can get histoplasmosis?

Anyone working at a job or present near activities where material contaminated with *H. capsulatum* becomes airborne can develop histoplasmosis if enough spores are inhaled. After an exposure, how ill a person becomes varies greatly and most likely depends on the number of spores inhaled and a person's age and susceptibility to the disease. The number of inhaled spores needed to cause disease is unknown. Children younger than 2 years of age, persons with compromised immune systems, and older persons, in particular those with underlying illnesses such as diabetes and chronic lung disease, are at increased risk for developing symptomatic histoplasmosis.

People with weakened immune systems are at greatest risk for developing severe and disseminated histoplasmosis. Included in this high-risk group are persons with AIDS or cancer and persons receiving cancer chemotherapy; high-dose, long-term steroid therapy; or other immuno-suppressive drugs.

Before 2000, a person could learn from a histoplasmin skin test whether he or she had been previously infected by *H. capsulatum*. However, the manufacturing of histoplasmin was discontinued in 2000, and the skin testing reagents were still unavailable in 2004. A previous infection can provide partial immunity to reinfection. Since a positive skin test does not mean that a person is completely immune to reinfection, appropriate exposure precautions should be taken regardless of a worker's past skin-test status whenever disturbances of materials that might be contaminated with *H. capsulatum* occur.

What is the treatment for histoplasmosis?

Mild cases of histoplasmosis are usually resolved without treatment. For severe cases, special anti-fungal medications are needed to arrest the disease. Disseminated histoplasmosis is fatal if untreated, but death can also occur in some patients even when medical treatment is received.

Where are *H. capsulatum* spores found?

H. capsulatum grows in soils throughout the world. In the United States, the fungus is endemic (more prevalent) and the proportion of people infected by *H. capsulatum* is higher in central and eastern states, especially along the Ohio and Mississippi River valleys. The fungus seems to grow best in soils having a high nitrogen content, especially those enriched with bat droppings or bird manure. Disturbances of contaminated material cause small *H. capsulatum* spores to become airborne or aerosolized. Once airborne, spores can easily be carried by wind currents over long distances.

How can someone know if soil or droppings are contaminated with *H. capsulatum* spores?

To learn whether soil or droppings are contaminated with *H. capsulatum* spores, samples must be collected and cultured. Presently, the method used to isolate *H. capsulatum* is expensive and requires several weeks to complete. If not enough samples are collected, small but highly contaminated areas can be overlooked. Until a less expensive and more rapid method is available, testing samples for *H. capsulatum* will continue to be impractical for most situations. Consequently, when thorough testing is not done, the safest approach is to assume soil in endemic regions and any accumulations of bat droppings or bird manure are contaminated with *H. capsulatum* and take appropriate exposure precautions.

What jobs and activities have risks for exposure to *H. capsulatum* spores?

Below is a partial list of occupations and hobbies with risks for exposure to *H. capsulatum* spores. Appropriate exposure precautions should be taken by these people and others whenever contaminated soil, bat droppings, or bird manure is disturbed.

- Bridge inspector or painter
- Chimney cleaner
- Construction worker
- Demolition worker
- Farmer
- Gardener
- Heating and air-conditioning system installer or service person
- Microbiology laboratory worker
- Pest control worker
- Restorer of historic or abandoned buildings
- Roofer
- Spelunker (cave explorer)

How can exposure to *H. capsulatum* be controlled and histoplasmosis prevented?

The best way to prevent exposures to *H. capsulatum* spores is to avoid situations where material that might be contaminated can become aerosolized and subsequently inhaled. This is especially important for persons with weakened immune systems.

Dust suppression methods, such as carefully wetting with a water spray, may be useful for reducing the amount of material aerosolized during an activity. For some activities, such as removing an accumulation of bat droppings or bird manure from an enclosed place such as an attic, wearing a NIOSH-approved respirator and other items of personal protective equipment may be needed to further reduce the risk of *H. capsulatum* exposure. However, only persons trained in the proper selection and use of personal protective equipment should undertake work where this equipment is needed

Disinfectants have occasionally been used to treat soil and accumulated bat manure when removal was impractical or as a precaution before a removal process was started. There is no product or chemical that is registered by the EPA that has the specific claim of being effective against *H. capsulatum*. A manufacturer of a product claiming to disinfect soil contaminated with *H. capsulatum* will have to meet the EPA's regulatory requirements and complete the registration process.

Where can I get more information about histoplasmosis?

This histoplasmosis fact sheet was prepared by the National Institute for Occupational Safety and Health (NIOSH) and the National Center for Infectious Diseases (NCID), both of the Centers for Disease Control and Prevention. For answers to other questions about histoplasmosis or histoplasmin skin-testing, please contact your physician, your local health department, or NCID in Atlanta, Georgia. NCID's Internet address is http://www.cdc.gov/ncidod/. For other questions about worker health and safety precautions during disturbances of soil, bat droppings, or bird manure that might be contaminated with *H. capsulatum* spores, call NIOSH in Cincinnati, Ohio, at (800) 356-4674.

HISTOPLASMOSIS

¿Qué es la histoplasmosis?

La histoplasmosis es una enfermedad infecciosa causada por la inhalación de esporas de un hongo llamado *Histoplasma capsulatum*. La histoplasmosis no es contagiosa; no puede ser transmitida de una persona o animal enfermo a alguien sano.

¿Cuales son los síntomas de la histoplasmosis?

La histoplasmosis afecta principalmente los pulmones y sus síntomas son muy variables. La gran mayoría de las personas infectadas son asintomáticas (no tienen efectos aparentes de enfermedad) o presentan síntomas tan leves que no requieren atención médica. Cuando hay síntomas, éstos generalmente empiezan 3 a 17 días después de la exposición, con un promedio de 10 días. La histoplasmosis puede aparecer como una enfermedad respiratoria leve tipo influenza y tiene una combinación de síntomas que incluyen decaimiento (sensación de enfermedad), fiebre, dolor en el pecho, tos seca o no productiva, dolor de cabeza, pérdida de apetito, disnea (dificultad para respirar), dolores musculares y de articulaciones, calofríos y ronquera. Una radiografía de tórax de una persona con histoplasmosis pulmonar aguda muestra con frecuencia una neumonitis desigual que se calcifica eventualmente. La enfermedad pulmonar crónica por histoplasmosis se parece a la tuberculosis y puede empeorar a través de los meses o años. La forma más severa y rara de esta enfermedad es la histoplasmosis diseminada, que involucra la invasión del hongo a otros órganos fuera de los pulmones.

¿Quién puede contraer histoplasmosis?

Cualquier persona que trabaje o esté presente cerca de actividades en donde el material contaminado con *H. capsulatum* se haga volátil, puede desarrollar histoplasmosis si inhala suficientes esporas. Después de una exposición, la severidad de la enfermedad es muy variable y probablemente dependa del número de esporas inhaladas y de la edad y susceptibilidad de la persona a contraer la enfermedad. El número de esporas que es necesario inhalar para contraer la enfermedad es desconocido. Los niños menores de dos años, las personas con sistemas inmunes comprometidos y los adultos mayores, en particular aquellos con enfermedades subyacentes tales como diabetes y enfermedad pulmonar crónica, tienen un mayor riesgo de desarrollar histoplasmosis sintomática.

Las personas con deficiencias del sistema inmune sufren mayor riesgo de desarrollar histoplasmosis severa y diseminada. Incluidos en este grupo de alto riesgo se encuentran las personas con SIDA o cáncer y las personas que están recibiendo quimioterapia, terapia con altas dosis de esteroides por tiempo prolongado o terapia con otros medicamentos inmunosupresores.

Antes del año 2000, una persona podía saber si había sido infectada previamente con *H. capsulatum* a través de una prueba cutánea con histoplasmina. Sin embargo, la fabricación de histoplasmina se descontinuó en 2000, y los reactivos para hacer la prueba cutánea seguían sin estar disponibles en el 2004. Una infección previa puede otorgar inmunidad parcial contra una reinfección. Dado que una prueba cutánea positiva no significa que una persona sea completamente inmune a una reinfección, deben ser adoptadas medidas apropiadas de protección contra la exposición. Estas medidas deberán ser adoptadas, independientemente de los resultados de la prueba cutánea, por aquellos trabajadores que manipulen materiales que puedan estar contaminados con *H. capsulatum*.

¿Cúal es el tratamiento de la histoplasmosis?

Los casos leves de histoplasmosis usualmente se resuelven sin tratamiento. Los casos severos requieren medicamentos especiales antihongos (fungicidas) para controlar la enfermedad. La histoplasmosis diseminada es mortal si no se trata, pero la muerte también puede ocurrir aún cuando se reciba tratamiento médico.

¿Dónde se encuentran las esporas de *H. capsulatum*?

El *H. capsulatum* se encuentra en suelos de todo el mundo. En los Estados Unidos, el hongo es endémico (más prevalente) y la proporción de gente infectada por *H. capsulatum* es mayor en los estados del este y el centro, sobre todo a lo largo de los valles de los ríos Ohio y Mississippi. El hongo parece crecer mejor en suelos con alto contenido de nitrógeno, especialmente aquellos enriquecidos con guano de murciélago o estiércol de pájaro. La manipulación de material contaminado hace que las pequeñas esporas de *H. capsulatum* se hagan volátiles o se conviertan en aerosol. Una vez volátiles, las esporas pueden ser fácilmente transportadas por corrientes de viento a grandes distancias.

¿Cómo se puede saber si el suelo o el guano están contaminadas con esporas de H. capsulatum?

Para saber si el suelo o el guano están contaminados con esporas de *H. capsulatum*, se deben tomar muestras para cultivo. Actualmente, el método usado para aislar *H. capsulatum* es caro y requiere varias semanas para completarlo. Si no se toman suficientes muestras, pueden ignorarse áreas pequeñas pero muy contaminadas. Hasta que exista un método más rápido y menos caro, el examen de muestras seguirá siendo poco práctico en la mayoría de las situaciones. En consecuencia, cuando no se hace un examen extensivo, el enfoque más seguro es asumir que el suelo en regiones endémicas y cualquier acumulación de guano de murciélago o estiércol de pájaro, están contaminados con *H. capsulatum* y, por lo tanto, tomar las medidas necesarias para prevenir la exposición.

¿Qué trabajos y actividades tienen riesgo de exposición a H. capsulatum?

A continuación hay una lista parcial de ocupaciones y pasatiempos que tienen riesgo de exposición a esporas de *H. capsulatum*. Estas personas deben tomar medidas adecuadas para prevenir la exposición siempre que se manipule suelo contaminado, guano de murciélago o estiércol de pájaro.

- Inspector o pintor de puentes
- Limpiador de chimeneas
- Trabajador de la construcción
- Trabajador de demolición
- Granjero, trabajador agrícola
- Jardinero
- Instalador o agente de servicio de sistemas de aire acondicionado y calefacción
- Trabajador de laboratorio microbiológico
- Trabajador de control de plagas
- Restaurador de edificios históricos o abandonados
- Trabajador de techos
- Explorador de cuevas

¿Cómo se puede controlar la exposición a H. capsulatum y prevenir la histoplasmosis?

La mejor forma de prevenir la exposición a las esporas de *H. capsulatum* es evitar aquellas situaciones donde materiales contaminados puedan hacerse volátiles y las esporas ser posteriormente inhaladas. Esto es importante sobre todo para aquellas personas con depresión del sistema inmune.

Los métodos de supresión de polvo, tal como humedecer cuidadosamente con un aspersor de agua, pueden ser útiles para reducir la cantidad de material que se volatiliza durante una actividad. Para algunas actividades, tales como remover una acumulación de guano de murciélago o estiércol de pájaro de un lugar cerrado, cómo un ático, se debe usar un respirador aprobado por NIOSH. Otros artículos de protección personal pueden ser necesarios para disminuir el riesgo de exposición a *H. capsulatum*. Sin embargo, sólo las personas capacitadas en la selección y el uso adecuados del equipo de protección personal deben llevar a cabo actividades donde este equipo sea requerido.

Ocasionalmente se han usado desinfectantes para tratar el suelo y la acumulación de guano de murciélago, cuando la remoción no es práctica, o como una precaución antes de iniciar el proceso de remoción. No existe producto o agente químico registrado por la EPA (Agencia de Protección Ambiental) que sea efectivo contra *H. capsulatum*. El fabricante de algún producto que afirme que desinfecta el suelo contaminado con *H. capsulatum* tendrá que cumplir con los requisitos regulatorios de la EPA y completar el proceso de registro.

¿Dónde se puede obtener más información sobre la histoplasmosis?

Esta hoja informativa sobre la histoplasmosis fue preparada por el Instituto Nacional de Salud y Seguridad Ocupacional (NIOSH) y el Centro Nacional de Enfermedades Infecciosas (NCID), ambos de los Centros de Control y Prevención de Enfermedades. Para respuestas a otras preguntas sobre histoplasmosis, por favor contacte a su médico, a su departamento de salud local, o al NCID en Atlanta, Georgia. La dirección de Internet del NCID es http://www.cdc.gov/ncidod/. Para otras consultas sobre la salud de los trabajadores y medidas de precaución a usar durante la manipulación de suelo, guano de murciélago o estiércol de pájaro potencialmente contaminados con esporas de *H. capsulatum*, llame a NIOSH en Cincinnati, Ohio, al teléfono (800) 356-4674.

2004